Clean Eating Alice

Everyday
Fitness

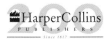

Thorsons
An imprint of HarperCollins*Publishers*
1 London Bridge Street
London SE1 9GF

www.harpercollins.co.uk

First published by Thorsons 2017

10 9 8 7 6 5 4 3 2 1

Photography © Philip Haynes
Food Photography © Martin Poole
Food Styling: Kim Morphew
Food Props Stylist: Wei Tang
Hair and make-up: Megan Koriat

A catalogue record of this book is available from the British Library

ISBN: 978-0-00-823800-1

Printed and bound by GPS Group

MIX
Paper from
responsible sources
FSC www.fsc.org **FSC˚ C007454**

FSC™ is a non-profit international organisation established to promote the responsible management of the world's forests. Products carrying the FSC label are independently certified to assure consumers that they come from forests that are managed to meet the social, economic and ecological needs of present and future generations, and other controlled sources.

Clean Eating Alice

Everyday Fitness

Train smart, eat well and
get the body you love

Thorsons

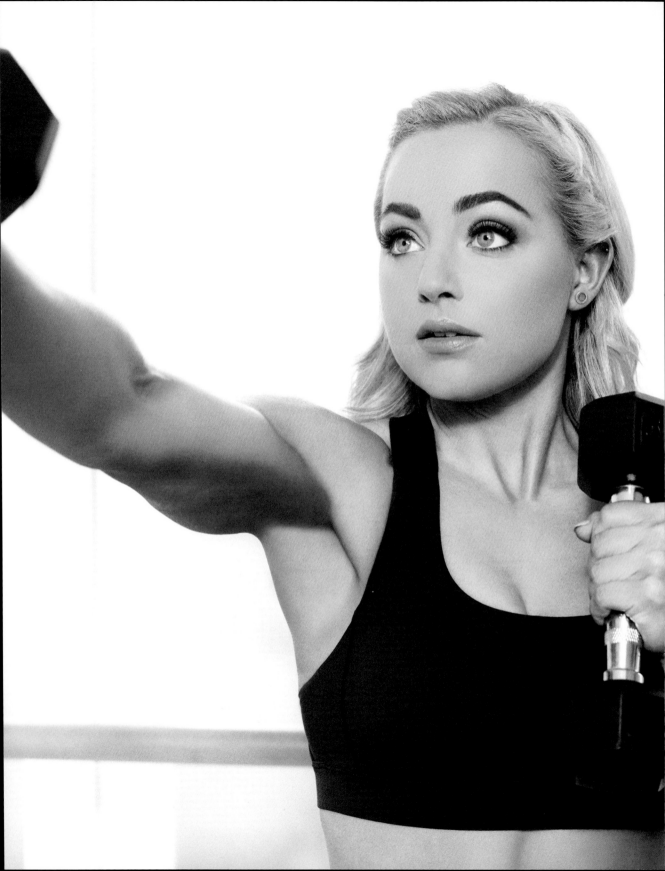

CONTENTS

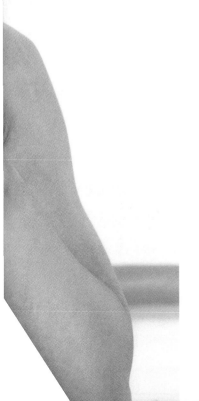

MY JOURNEY TO FIT

The first thing I want to say to you all is a big 'Thank you' for buying this book. With the abundance of information, workout videos and internet gurus out there now, and the fitness bubble ever expanding with no sign of a slowdown, I appreciate your decision to read this book and take control of your journey. That journey begins *right now*.

For those who don't know much about me, I am Alice, the girl behind the Instagram blog Clean Eating Alice, which I began in 2014 while studying musical theatre at university. It was my private page which I started in order to document my own personal health kick, after reaching what felt like rock bottom with how I felt about my physique, and how my own eating habits had spiralled out of control. I don't think my story is any different to those of so many people, but at the time, and surrounded by friends who could eat whatever they wanted and not gain a pound, I felt completely alone. This led me to reach out and start my Instagram blog, and I began to post pictures of every meal I was eating each day, to encourage a sense of pride in my meals and develop a better relationship with food, which at that point was incredibly poor. The page also acted as perfect motivation to keep momentum with

this journey, instead of falling off the diet wagon – which I'd done so many times previously, trying various fad diets and fitness trends.

Over a period of a few months (and as I got to grips with how to actually take a good photo), what had once been a very small private space I posted on each day with very little traction soon started to grow in audience numbers. Within a few more months I realised that there was a whole community of people who were in a similar position to me, and who had turned to social media as a sort of support network to help them keep motivated and progress with their own goals. Where once you might have wandered down to your local community Weight Watchers group as a means of interacting with others on a similar path to yours, the internet now provided a community larger than I could even fathom, of like-minded, motivated women who wanted to share and grow

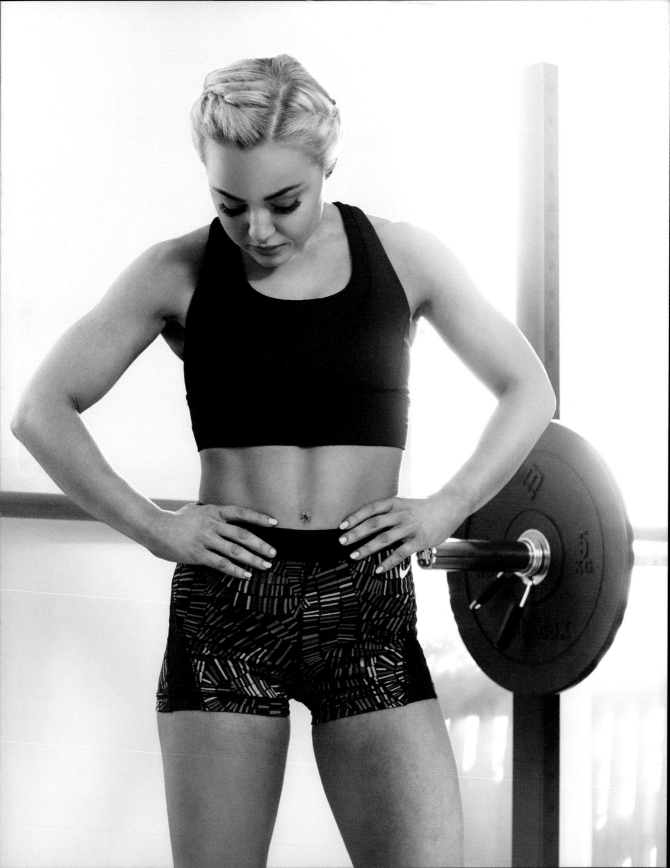

together, with daily encouragement and swapping of recipes, gym advice and more. As my journey progressed, this increase in followers escalated, and it wasn't long before I was interacting with both men and women each day, learning from others and sharing experiences.

Since those early days of blogging, I feel I have transformed myself both inside and out, with the help of this incredible online community. I have totally addressed and overcome what seemed like an endless cycle of bingeing and then overly restricting my food intake, and I have spent the past two years working to gain strength and build lean muscle in the gym. As cringey as it may sound, I honestly don't feel I would be the person I am today without having experienced the journey I have been on, including highs and lows – of both there have been many. I have learned a hell of a lot, had the opportunity to work with some incredibly inspiring people and achieved things I thought only existed in my wildest dreams. But, no matter how exciting my success may be, my ethos remains the same as the day I started, and continues to be uncompromising. It is this ethos and passion for what I do that has driven me to write this book for you.

It is important to begin by crediting the majority of my transformation to the change in my nutrition, rather than the training that I later embarked on, which is why I've included a range of recipes to inspire you to take charge of your diet. I can't impress enough on you how strongly I believe that diet and exercise go hand in hand, and neglecting one for the other will ultimately have a negative effect on achieving your goals. From my own personal journey, I saw first-hand how my poor nutrition caused me to dramatically gain weight, despite the fact that I was at dance college exercising more than ever. That is why my first

two books have focused predominantly on diet, and encouraging you all to create delicious recipes that draw you away from restrictive diets, and instead place a focus on encouraging a balanced and inclusive relationship with food. However, while of course I do admit that food certainly came first in terms of my own transformation, I truly believe my physique change would not have been as dramatic as it was, nor as sustainable and maintainable as it has been, without the incorporation of exercise into my lifestyle. And when I say exercise, I don't mean what I perceived to be exercise … mind-numbingly boring, facing-a-blank-wall treadmill work. I mean finding a way of exercise that I enjoyed, and that I was able to progress with, using goal-setting and different techniques to keep up. And, most importantly, beginning to see that exercise didn't have to be that awful thing we all know we should do, but that we dread none the less. It was when I married these two components together that I achieved the most successful outcome, and the best progression.

While you'll never hear the phrase 'bikini body' exit my mouth, I often find my clients are at their most motivated during the summer months. At this time of the year the weather is warming up, we're beginning to ditch our winter layers and the prospect of a beach holiday is just around the corner, which often provides the perfect inspiration to kickstart your fitness journey. It's not about fitting a 'bikini body' stereotype or reaching a number on the scales – the thing that embarking on this fitness journey is hopefully going to change is how you *feel* in that bikini.

In all three of my books I have talked about how my own journey fell into place when I combined hard work in the gym with consistent healthy and nutritious eating, as well as a whole lot

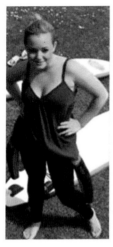
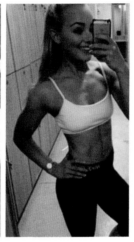
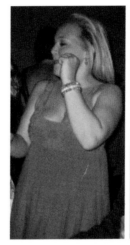
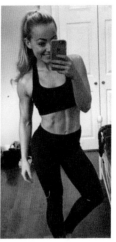
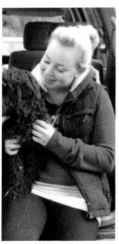
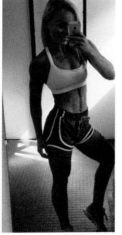
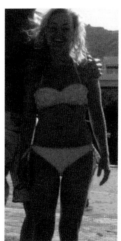
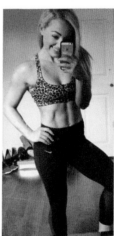

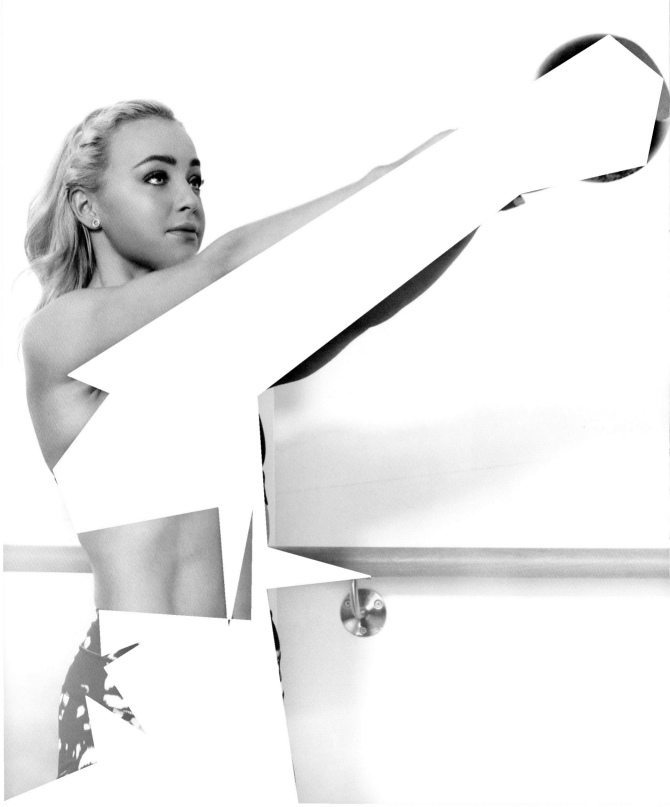

of self-motivation and self-love. I was then able to shed the pounds I'd tried so hard to lose on every fad diet going. This book will hopefully fall into your lap at a time when the weather is nice and the days feel longer, and you've got enough time before the summer holidays kick in to really build some lean muscle, while losing body fat. That's not to say you're only creating a 'summer body' – you all know that I am the antithesis of 'quick fixes' – but using this increase in motivation to eat well and move more will set you on your way to an all-round leaner, fitter and healthier you!

So here we are, two years later, and with what I've just shared in mind, I've felt so incredibly passionate about writing this book to hopefully help some of you to also embrace good nutrition and exercise and create happy and healthy lifestyles for yourselves. As a now practising personal trainer with a breadth of clients, I've honed my craft towards helping not only myself but also my clients to achieve their goals, and finding the best and most effective ways to do this. But let me stop you right there if what you think I want you to achieve is rippling abs and a muscular physique. I am fully aware that some may see me as 'fitspo', but I'm not a fan of that label. For so long I thought my identity lay in the fact that I was a girl with abs, and quite honestly it didn't make me feel great. What made me feel amazing – and what I wish you to get from this book – was to find a way to love and embrace my body. To move more, in whatever way makes you happy, to feel the sense of freedom that comes from taking control of your life and body and to celebrate what you are every day. That is what has made me truly happy, and what I hope will help you to feel the same. And on that note, so begins this book. It's a journey, and I am with you every step of the way.

CLIENT TESTIMONIALS:

Over my time as a personal trainer I have accumulated a range of different clients, all with varying needs and goals. This has allowed me to be challenged, not only as a trainer but as a person, too. Being a personal trainer for me isn't just about providing someone with an hour of exercise for the week. I hope to deliver my clients so much more than that. Throughout this book you will read a few of my clients' testimonials, sharing their experience of training with me. I've included these to show my credibility beyond just being a girl who posts exercise videos on Instagram. I take my job incredibly seriously and I am so lucky to have the opportunity to help people to achieve their goals in the healthiest, happiest way possible, just as I did.

MY JOURNEY TO FIT: HOW I BEGAN TRAINING

I was never the sporty kid at school. While all my friends happily wore their knee-high socks and inserted mouth-guards to head up to the cold playing fields for lacrosse, I hobbled around the changing rooms continuing to pretend I had an injury in order to get out of PE yet again.

It wasn't that I was necessarily bad at sport – I was a keen dancer out of school hours – I just dreaded the very thought of it. I didn't apply myself, therefore I never really got to see what I was capable of. As I entered the sixth form we were given various exercise options within our allocated physical-education slots, with time spent in our school gym being one of them. As every other sport choice looked abysmal to me, I chose this option, and so began my gym journey.

The gym for me is an anomaly when it comes to exercise. With most activities we are taught or coached in how to do them in a controlled environment, whether it be at school or at various clubs. Yet with the gym, unless you pay for a personal trainer, there is no real guidance. This means, at worst, anyone can walk in, start lifting weights and potentially do themselves serious damage. At best they will achieve very little for lack of knowing what to do. Because of this, my first ever gym session was spent wandering around, aimlessly examining each piece of equipment, followed by about ten minutes on the treadmill, ten on the cross-trainer, and a few sit-ups for good measure. This format then became my standard gym routine, and I continued this way for the rest of my time in sixth form.

As mentioned before, that didn't mean that I didn't do any activity at all aside from my half-hearted gym sessions. I loved dancing and would attend ballet and jazz classes after school. These sessions inspired me to want to follow a career in theatre. I'd always loved performing, and knew that while I enjoyed my academic studies I also loved the idea of being able to follow my true passion when I left school. By the time I finished sixth form I'd decided that I wanted to seriously pursue this as a career, and after a terrifying and intense load of auditions for theatre schools, I won a place at the brilliant Bird College.

Once I started college, I quickly realised that I was physically different from a lot of the other girls in my year. I don't have a typical dancer's body, and where lots of girls in my year were tall with long legs, I found myself standing at five-foot one, slightly chubby and severely lacking in leg length. As the three-year course began I would be in a leotard and tights all day, feeling totally uncomfortable and comparing myself to everyone else in the room instead of concentrating on my own studies. I found my passion for my course dwindled as I became self-conscious about my body and started to doubt my abilities. As time passed it was clear that I experienced total regression with my dance training and it was having an impact on my physique.

I was eating more than ever, all the wrong things, and slowly putting on weight. This was a two-part reaction: I subconsciously increased my caloric intake as, in my eyes, I was exercising a lot and therefore could eat whatever I wanted, and I found comfort in the food I was eating, to make myself feel better about the situation I was in.

The real wake-up call came for me at the end of my first year at college. We had end-of-year assessments in all dance and theatre disciplines, from ballet to jazz to tap, etc. It's safe to say that I did pretty poorly across the board, with the recurring phrase of 'lacking in strength' being written on my reports. It was around this time that the penny really dropped for me. I'd spent so long dreaming about being on the stage, performing for a living, and I was letting that dream slowly slip away due to my inability to apply myself to my training. Instead of focusing on my strengths, I fixated on my weaknesses and therefore allowed myself to get stuck in a mindset of not being good enough. I decided at this point that strength would become my strength. I could never work miracles and suddenly grow a few extra inches, and even with all the stretching in the world I would never have long legs, but I could be the strongest dancer, strong in body and in mind, and it was this moment that spurred me to re-enter the gym.

At this point I was entering into my second year of college, and moved into a flat conveniently located two minutes away from my local gym, so there were no excuses. I started to go after college a few days a week, picking up where I left off with my 20 minutes of random cardiovascular exercise, followed by a few sit-ups, and maybe a plank here and there. Of course I had the best intentions with every session, but I soon found myself incredibly bored of running while staring at a blank wall, no matter how good my workout playlist was. On one such gym visit I

got talking to a personal trainer, and he suggested I try incorporating some weight-training into my sessions. As I had no prior knowledge, he showed me a few basic weight-training exercises – from coaching my squat to a few moves on the cable machine. So began my weight-training journey.

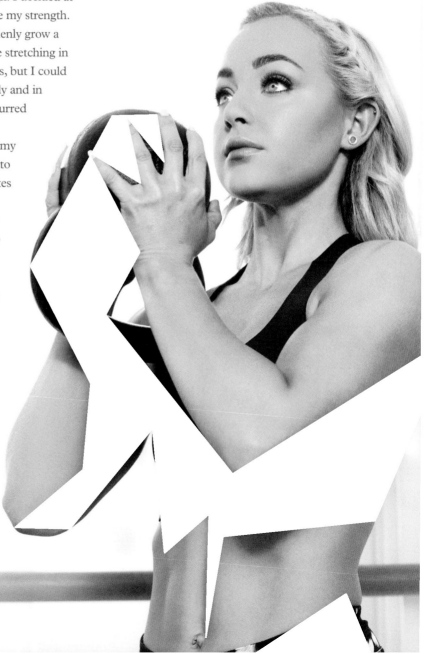

MY JOURNEY TO FIT:
DISCOVERING WEIGHT-TRAINING

From this point onwards I developed a real interest in and passion for weight-training. I loved the diversity of each gym session, which was a million miles away from the same old repetitive treadmill slog. In the very beginning I really focused my training around the small handful of exercises that I had been shown. Without knowing it, this was the best foundation I could have been given, as it allowed me to build strength and confidence in the major compound lifts such as squats, presses and rows in their most basic form, before I added anything fancy or any accessory work to my routine.

At this very initial stage of my journey I was given a very old but very useful guide to lifting by the same personal trainer, which showed all the various muscle groups, and different exercises for each, ranging from the basic compound moves with explanations, and a few more isolation exercises, too. After a short while I began incorporating these into my gym sessions. From day one of exploring this way of training I felt my motivation increase dramatically. Suddenly my exercise was challenging my body in a completely different way and therefore became

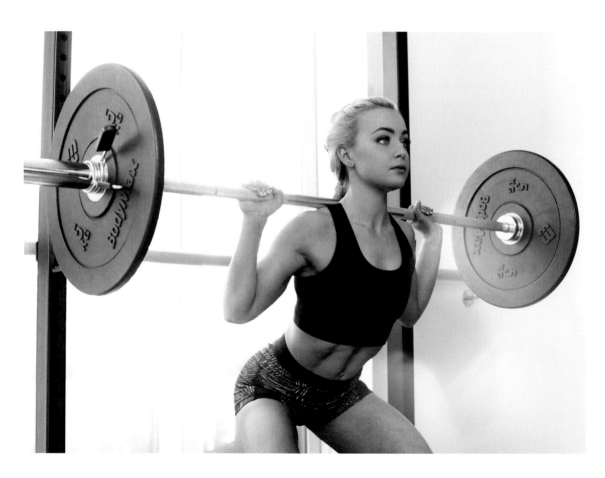

really interesting, and I enjoyed the experience of trying new exercises and expanding my exercise vocabulary. I gradually grew my abilities within the gym and, slowly but surely, gained confidence in my technique. One thing I loved was how it became an incredibly empowering experience to venture into the once male-dominated weights area of the gym and know exactly what to do.

Girls and weights had previously been a complete taboo, and it was a rare sight to catch a girl in the weights section. That has all changed in the last few years, and I now felt completely at ease and confident enough to hold my own and know what I was doing in such a testosterone-fuelled environment.

My training when I first started was structured a little differently from how I now train, and it's important to emphasise to you that I didn't become an expert overnight. I really make clear to all my new clients, who mostly have very little experience of lifting, that it is so important to properly invest in building solid foundations from which to progress, instead of jumping the gun and potentially doing serious harm through injury. I am not ashamed of the fact that I spent the whole of the first year that I trained focusing on a very small handful of exercises such as a chest press, a squat and a deadlift, as I didn't feel confident or able to go beyond these core moves. That being said, what I did do was progressively gain strength in all of these exercises, slowly building up the amount of weight that I was lifting each week, and it was through this that I really started to notice changes in my physique. This is a sentiment I reiterate throughout this entire book. I want this to be accessible and achievable, while challenging enough to create physical change and help you achieve your goals. Just as I took a slow and

steady pace to gain confidence with my training, I urge you to move at a pace that is right for you and your body.

Fast-forward to now; I have never completely lost passion for my training, and while of course I can experience lapses in motivation, I've used these to slightly change tack, try something new or reassess my goals. However, I do continue to strength-train four to five times a week, with a renewed knowledge and understanding of both my body and the way I enjoy training. I decided I wanted to gain my Level 3 personal-training qualifications to further my passion for helping others to understand the benefits of weight-training. Since qualifying I have worked with a whole host of different clients with varying abilities; this has further challenged me to develop and refine my skills as a personal trainer. But it has also enabled me to be empathetic and understanding of what it feels like to be at the very start of a fitness journey. I know what it feels like to be at rock bottom with body confidence, and I try to change a judgemental mentality in any of my clients before they start training with me.

Through working face-to-face with clients, I have developed a particular love for helping women to become strong, body-confident individuals, and I hope that through this book I can pass this message on to even more of you, to help as many of you as possible achieve lasting health and happiness.

As mentioned, for the past three years, since discovering strength-training, I have never lost passion for it, and continue to train in this way four to five times a week. That being said, I've worked incredibly hard to refine my technique, expand my knowledge and improve in all areas of my training. I continue to set new goals each month to help keep my training varied.

MY EXERCISE ETHOS

In my opinion, exercise is the most untapped resource for improving general happiness. My favourite saying is 'strong in mind, strong in body' – and I aim to help you achieve both.

- Exercise should be accessible to ALL, no matter what level of experience, age, shape or size.

- It should be simple. There is no point making something so hard or confusing that you can't actually do it, be that with exercise or nutrition. For me, simplicity is key, and nailing the basics is the best way to build strong foundations from which you can then progress.

- It should be progressive. With any exercise programme or regime, there needs to be the ability to see improvement. With all the exercises in this book there is the potential to progress or regress depending on your ability, and a full explanation is included as to how to personalise your own programme and track your improvement. This is really important to help you see encouraging results that will keep you committed and focused.

- It should be fun. Nobody likes slogging away at something they absolutely loathe. Me especially! While I'm not saying that every gym session is going to be a fun-filled hour of easiness, there are ways and means to creating a positive and enjoyable environment. Use good gym playlists, plan some delicious post-workout food or buddy up with a friend to make training as enjoyable as possible.

- It should be efficient. Workouts don't have to be hours long to be effective, and often with training it is a case of quality over quantity. I don't expect anyone to have hours to spend on their exercise routine, therefore intensity is key, and inputting the right amount into your session is far more beneficial than an hour of what I describe as 'equipment hopping'.

- It should be realistic. While your training is important in creating physical change, it also begins and ends with mindset – you are never going to achieve all that you want to if you don't have the motivation to get yourself to the gym in the first place. Don't overdo it on the ambition front – set small and achievable targets that mean something to you. Don't worry about what you think you should be doing or what everyone else is up to – it's about what works for you. The truth is that if you set yourself impossible tasks, your relationship with fitness will be a flash in the pan rather than something you nurture and build. The worst thing anyone can feel in relation to fitness is guilt or anxiety. Be kind to yourself.

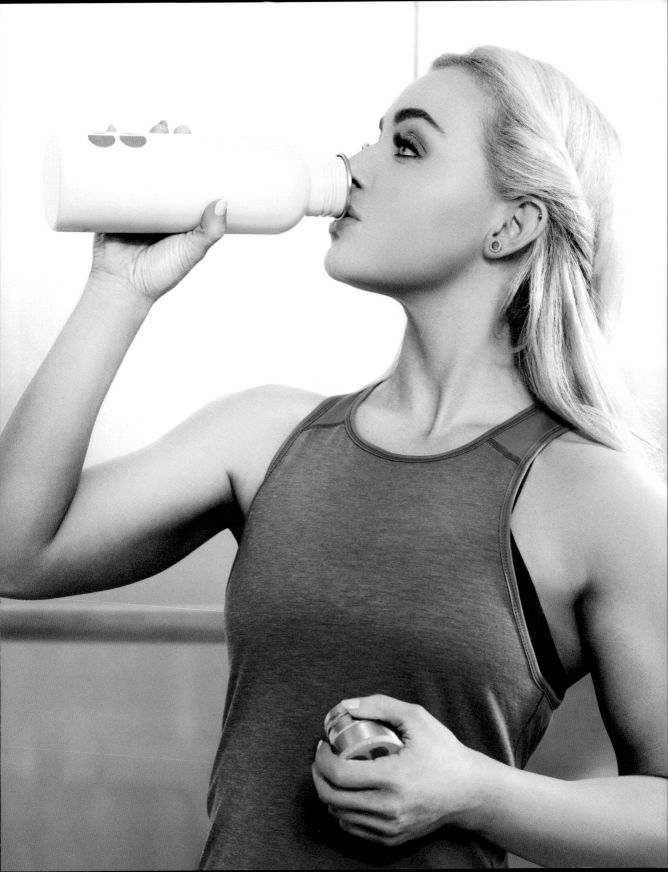

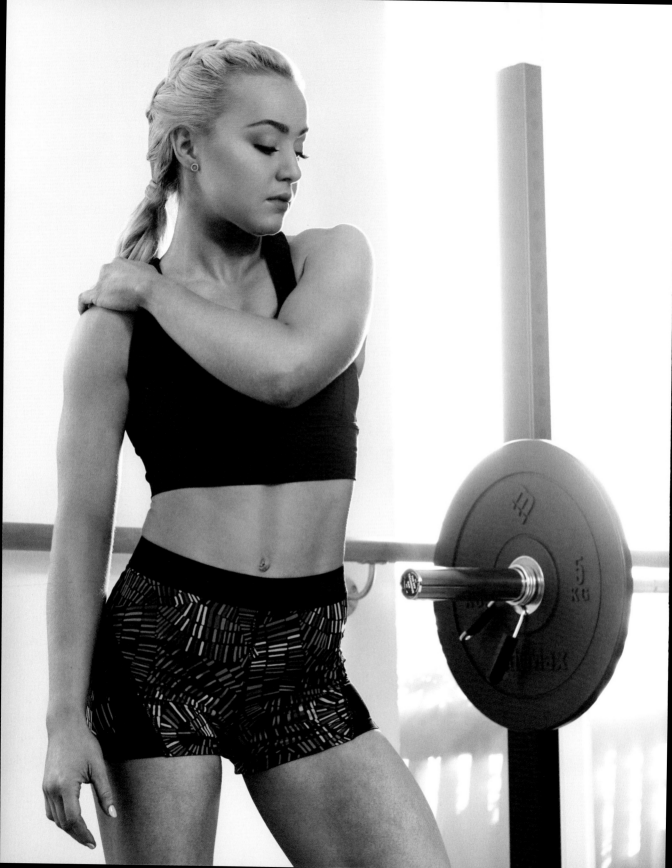

MY EXERCISE ETHOS: ACCESSIBLE EXERCISE

I have an uncompromising opinion that exercise should be accessible to all. Whether you're a busy mum, a nightshift worker or a complete beginner – whoever you are, exercise shouldn't be seen as an unattainable ideal that can never be achieved, or as something that takes an enormous amount of time and dedication to fit into your everyday life.

There is no right or wrong way to incorporate exercise into your lifestyle, nor is there one way that achieves better results than another. We all have our likes and dislikes, and it is absolutely OK to not like weight-training, just as it is OK to enjoy classes such as zumba or getting into the pool for a swim. What I really want to impress upon you is that this book is here to encourage you to look past aesthetic goals, which is something I reiterate to all my clients. This book is here to show you functional fitness that is designed to improve both muscular and cardiovascular health, not for a short-term gain but longevity, improved overall health and, ultimately and most importantly, happiness.

MY EXERCISE ETHOS: FINDING THE BALANCE

As with anything that makes us feel good, we can often go full circle with exercise. From it being the part of our week we absolutely loathe, suddenly the high of endorphins and escapism that our allocated exercise slot provides us can become all too addictive. For me it's important,

as with everything in life, to find the right balance with exercise. It shouldn't be used as a tool to compensate for a poor diet – one of my favourite sayings still remains true, that you can't out-train a bad diet. Nor should it be something that you, at any point, associate with guilt if you miss a workout, or life takes over and you fall off-track.

As with maintaining a good diet, flexibility is key to long-term sustainability, and that is what I hope this book will provide.

MY EXERCISE ETHOS: THE DANGERS OF OVERTRAINING

- Increased cortisol (stress hormone) levels
- Poor-quality sleep
- Reduced performance
- Bingeing on exercise, and the guilt attached if training sessions are missed
- Increased muscular pain, as opposed to just muscle soreness

All of the above are things that I encounter on a regular basis with my own clients and people I come into contact with in the fitness industry. As the wellness bubble has boomed, it's suddenly become acceptable and almost celebrated to submit our bodies to continuous strain, with very little chance for adequate recovery.

HOW TO USE EVERYDAY FITNESS

I have designed this book to help you on your fitness journey, with health and happiness at the forefront of what I want you to get from this guide.

With this in mind, it's important that we look at all aspects of training: this will include the motivation needed to help kickstart your routine, tips on how you maintain it, help and advice with goal-setting, tracking your progress, recovery and, of course, educating you on your nutrition. What you fuel your body with before, during and after training underpins what you will get out of your exercise programme. I want this book to be your one-stop bible for an accessible, easy and effective way of training, allowing me to be your own pocket personal trainer at no extra cost!

With such a wealth of information now available via the internet, it's so important to understand that there really is no right or wrong way to exercise, and obsessing over the minute details of your training may lead you to lose sight of the bigger picture and what you want to achieve. For that reason I have tried not to bombard you with an excessive number of exercises, but instead have focused on helping you to build solid foundations in your training, from which you can then progress and expand your exercise vocabulary. The beauty of this book is

that I want you to have the ability to personalise and tailor these workouts to your own goals and needs. As with nutrition, there really is no one-size-fits-all when it comes to fitness, and trying to be everything to everyone would be a pointless exercise. *Everyday Fitness* is about empowering you to learn how to slot fitness into a routine that suits your lifestyle and, most importantly, your goals. I want you to identify your goals, set them, smash them and be encouraged to just get better and better. For me, when writing all of my books it has never been about telling you to do as I do; I don't believe in pushing my routine onto others or implying my way is the only way to get fit and feel great. I do what works for ME and it has taken me a long time, and a lot of hard work, to get to the place where I feel fully confident in my own goals and abilities, and where I feel I know my own body. It is a cliché to use the word 'journey', but that's what it is – a path of trial and error, and not being afraid to try new things as you search for the best way to identify what you want for your body and mind. Then the challenge is to make it happen.

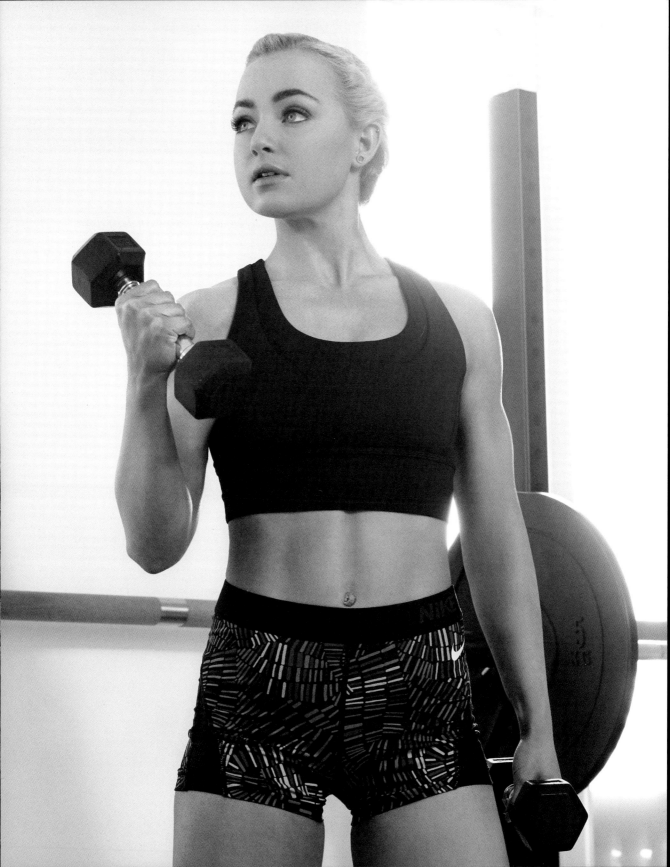

you are equipped with the most solid foundations from which you can then progress with your training. This is to ensure that you not only feel ready and able to step into the gym environment with absolute confidence, but also have the ability to execute each exercise with correct form to avoid injury or repetitive strain.

Ultimately, I want you to be able to use this book as a tool to suit your needs. Not your friend's, not your sister's or your work colleague's, but YOUR needs. I only hope that you can ignite your passion to incorporate fitness into your lifestyle with the correct vocabulary and know-how for the most effective training possible.

There is no magic wand, but in my experience we feel most motivated with our training when there is a plan in place, goals are set and we know what we are doing within each session. This not only makes for the most effective training, but also ensures that you are able to progress safely and at your own pace, and you can grow in confidence with all the basic exercises, creating strong foundations to then move on to more advanced strength-training.

But that is not my only goal. Our bodies are the vehicles that carry us through life. They need good fuel, in the form of solid nutrition, but they also need movement to keep them functioning to the best of their ability. If we left a car sitting on the drive for a few months, chances are it might be a little rusty when we then went to drive it. The same can be said for our bodies. If we don't move outside of our everyday functional movements, the chances are that our mobility will decrease and regress to the small amount of repetitive movements we do every day: things like sitting down, walking up stairs and picking things up off the ground. A very well-known movement practitioner once stated that, 'Learning to move correctly in the gym is like

Included in the exercise part of this book are three sections of varying workouts, designed to give you as much flexibility with your training as possible, and help you find a balance to slot fitness into your life however you see fit. I speak to so many people who for different reasons choose to work out at home, and it is my intention to provide you with as much useful guidance as I can for how to achieve a good workout in the comfort of your own home. Another issue with exercise is how to fit it into the day, with time constraints often being one of the main contributing factors as to why people don't – or aren't able to – exercise. For this reason I have included the HIIT workouts, designed to help those with limited time still achieve an efficient workout without impacting too much on their day.

Finally, the last exercise section of this book will, I hope, speak to those who wish to explore the gym environment and perhaps try their hand at strength-training. These workouts will be slightly longer, to allow for effective mobilisation and warmed-up muscles pre-workout, followed by training sessions that focus on specific muscle groups. It is so important that within this book learning to read and write in school, in that you get a formal education and become fluent. The bad news is that you're going to have to invest some time to learn the basics. The good news is that it's never too late to start.'

Within this book you will be shown the best and most effective exercises to create a lean and fit body, with functionality and building proper foundations at the heart of all you'll learn. While aiming for aesthetics can often seem like the most desirable goal, it's time to see past that, and train smart for long-term health.

CLIENT TESTIMONIAL: MARSHA

Since training with Alice, I've seen my body completely change as I've got stronger and leaner. Alice is always smiling, and makes every session exciting and different so that I never get bored or dread my training sessions. She is a pleasure to be trained by, and I would highly recommend her as a trainer to anyone!

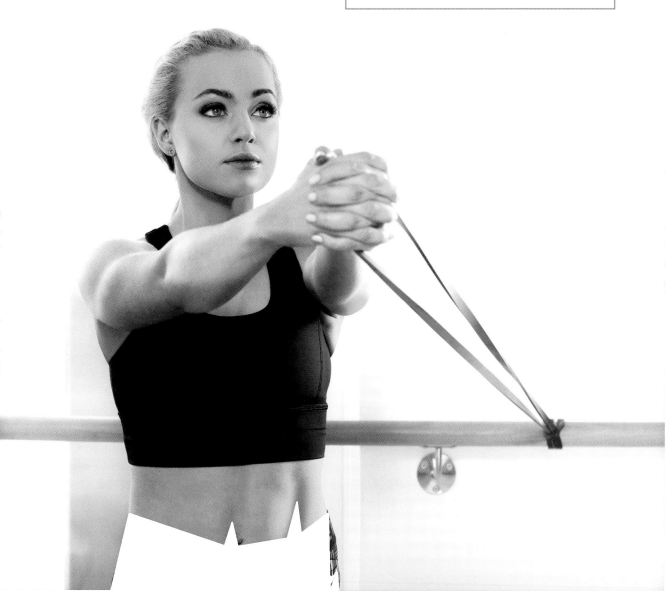

KICKSTARTING YOUR FITNESS JOURNEY

MOTIVATION

Before you begin any fitness journey, you need the motivation to actually start. For some, this can be as simple as waking up one day and deciding to try something new, while for others it sometimes calls for a little bit of assistance to help get them on their way. While I don't hold the secret to endless motivation, I want to share with you some of the ways in which I kickstart and maintain it with my own training.

When I first began training I trained in a completely different way to how I train now. That's not to say either is right or wrong, but my motivation and goals have shifted, my schedule has increased and therefore I've had to make adjustments to how I exercise. In addition, throughout this period of time my motivation stimulus has varied dramatically, from photoshoots to wanting to get stronger, to simply training as a social activity. It's important to understand that it is OK to have days or weeks of little if any motivation to get up and get active. The important thing is to incorporate these tips and tricks if you find yourself stuck in a rut, and to constantly equip you to adapt and evolve your training stimulus as you grow in confidence and ability.

Before I start training any of my clients, one of the first things I do is try to tap into what I think is motivating them from the outset – that way I get to know how I will keep their enthusiasm and commitment going long term. Often we, as personal trainers, spend time refining what clients 'think' will get them going, only to find that their longer-term goals can be confused and unclear. Before we can identify what those goals are, we have to find out what sparks up the individual and what will get them through the early stages.

HAVE A GOAL

I will cover goal-setting in more detail later in the book, as I feel it's such an important tool to get you going, but the word can often seem quite vague. I am a huge advocate of making goals gym-based and to do with your mental thought process, rather than just focusing on an aesthetic change, which can often lead to obsessing over body hang-ups. For more help on this, see page 34.

HAVE A PLAN

I hope that what this book gives you is structure to your training. In my own experience there is nothing worse than walking into the gym, or deciding you want to work out, and then not quite knowing what to do. I've wasted many a gym session wandering aimlessly from exercise to exercise in a half-hearted manner as I try to piece together a workout – this is a sure way to leave you feeling incredibly demotivated. Within this book you will find workouts that will give a consistent structure to your training so that you can know exactly what you are doing before you begin training, and have the ability to maintain consistency in your training so that you can track your progress easily. Simply having a plan in place and knowing what you are going to do before you set out to train can make all the difference to the outcome of your session.

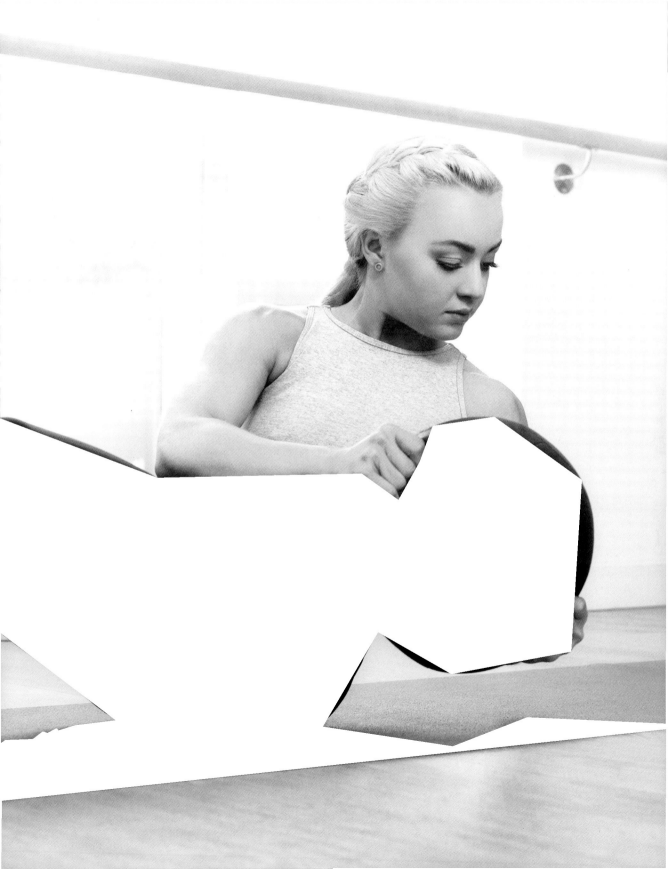

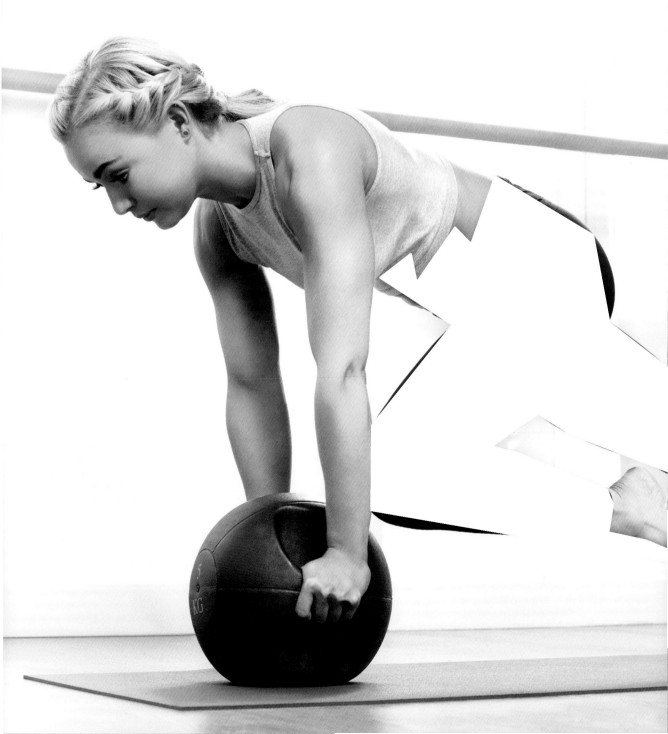

CLIENT TESTIMONIAL: LYDIA

I was completely lost before reaching out to Alice for help; my bad relationship with food and my body, alongside a chronic disease, had me interpreting things in a really negative way. Alice is an inspiration, both in the journey she has taken but also by being kind and passionate when I needed it the most. It's easy when it comes to food and exercise for personal trainers, magazines and diet books to use negativity, deprivation and guilt to try to influence the lifestyle choices we make; it's much harder to stay focused and find the positivity in transforming our lives and loving the journey. Alice continues to help me become the positive, healthy, happy person I want to be. Sessions with Alice don't take time away from my life, they add so much to it. I feel very lucky to have such a wonderful influence in a personal trainer and friend.

DON'T OVERDO IT

While we all set out on a fitness journey with the best intentions, it can often be the case that we start off on the wrong foot at a million miles an hour, perhaps training excessively, which then leads to an unsustainable training schedule. As the feel-good factor of the first few weeks of training begins to wear off, it is then easy to lose momentum, and in my experience it's at this point that a lot of people give up. While it is totally OK to be ambitious with your training, there is a fine line between this and then overdoing it by potentially overtraining, which will be to the detriment of your long-term motivation. The

saying 'don't run before you can walk' rings true here, and is something I impress on all my clients.

Starting with baby steps, slowly build up your body's tolerance to training so that you can have a clear and sustainable exercise regime that doesn't burn you out in the first week. Perhaps aim for two or three training sessions in the first week and then gradually build on this week on week until you reach a level that is challenging yet sustainable for you, and that you are able to realistically fit into your lifestyle.

BUDDY UP

While it's not always achievable to train with someone all the time, sometimes partnering up with a friend or training partner can be the best way to kickstart your motivation. If you've agreed to train together, you are less likely to bail on a friend than you are if you were training alone and there is no one to make you accountable. In addition to this, others always train slightly differently from you, with perhaps different exercises or different ways of doing similar exercises, giving you a great way to learn and breathe new life into your own training.

If you struggle to find someone at your gym or if you work out from home, this is the perfect opportunity to perhaps seek out an online training buddy, or simply use social media to find others with similar interests to you. I have personally reaped the benefits of the online fitness community, and relied on the support that I've received from it during the beginning phase of my journey, and I am a huge advocate of using social media to kickstart motivation.

I found in the early days of my blogging and fitness journey that reaching out to people in a similar situation to me helped to reduce the feeling of isolation that I sometimes encountered. I was fortunate enough to have amazing and supportive friends throughout my journey, but that didn't mean they were interested in training with me, or eating the way I did. This meant that, while they were incredibly supportive, I used the online community to discuss and interact with others on various topics, instead of boring my housemates with each of my meals or gym sessions. It is amazing how much motivation I used to (and still do) get from a positive comment left underneath a post I have uploaded – if someone likes a recipe I leave or tells me that one of my videos was the inspiration to get them back to the gym or to try to lift a heavier weight. That buzz I get comes from the knowledge that I am helping someone, but also from knowing I am part of a bigger community that understands how I think and feel about food and fitness.

Finding your sort of people is essential to staying focused and also to having others you can celebrate your achievements with – no matter how big or small.

TRY SOMETHING NEW

This book isn't just for people at the beginning of their fitness journey, as even those who've trained for years can go through lapses in motivation. It's impossible to maintain high levels of enthusiasm with the same style of training for prolonged periods of time, without experiencing some lapses. While this is totally normal, and can be worked through a lot of the time, it can also be good to use this opportunity to try something different.

When it comes to weight-training, something I've personally done to keep my motivation high is to set myself the challenge of a certain number of new techniques within a designated time-frame. For example, I challenge myself by trying different power-lifting techniques, over purely bodybuilding-style training. This encourages me to use my body and my strength in a completely different way from how I once used to, and gives me a new focus and new-found drive to get to the gym and train. The variety was just what I needed to reconnect and feel like I was doing something fresh. In reality I was still lifting, but I was just challenging myself in a completely different way.

Simply switching up your training stimulus can help reignite your passion for keeping active. This could be as simple as trying a new class, a new lift in the gym or a new team sport, taking a friend and seeing how much they get out of something you've been doing for a while and have maybe lost the joy for. I hope this book can also be the perfect stimulus to help you try something that is perhaps different from your usual training, and provide you with some much-needed motivation.

GEEK OUT

Since beginning my blog, I have made it my mission to ensure I am clued up with both my training and nutrition to ensure that I know why I am doing what I am doing.

After qualifying as a Level 3 personal trainer, I've attended seminars, listened to podcasts and read and invested time in training with or following people who I feel I have something to learn from.

I am currently doing an AFN-certified nutrition course with the Nutrition Academy to help further my nutritional knowledge and am taking a course with the UK Strength and Conditioning Association, as well as aiming to get my Level 4 personal-training qualifications this year. I'm not saying that any of you need to invest as heavily in your education, but I've personally found that just expanding my knowledge gives me the ability to make better decisions for myself, rather than following what someone else has done.

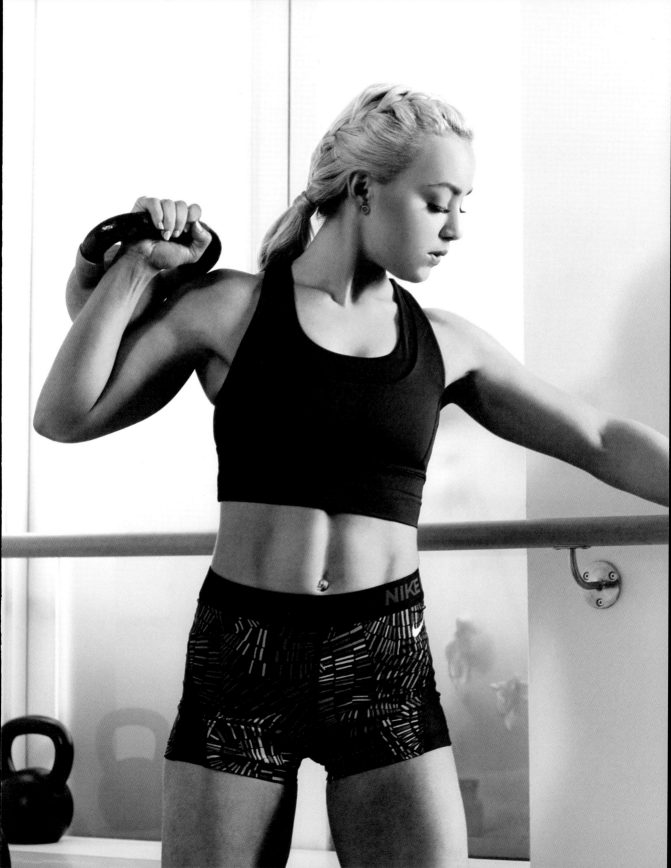

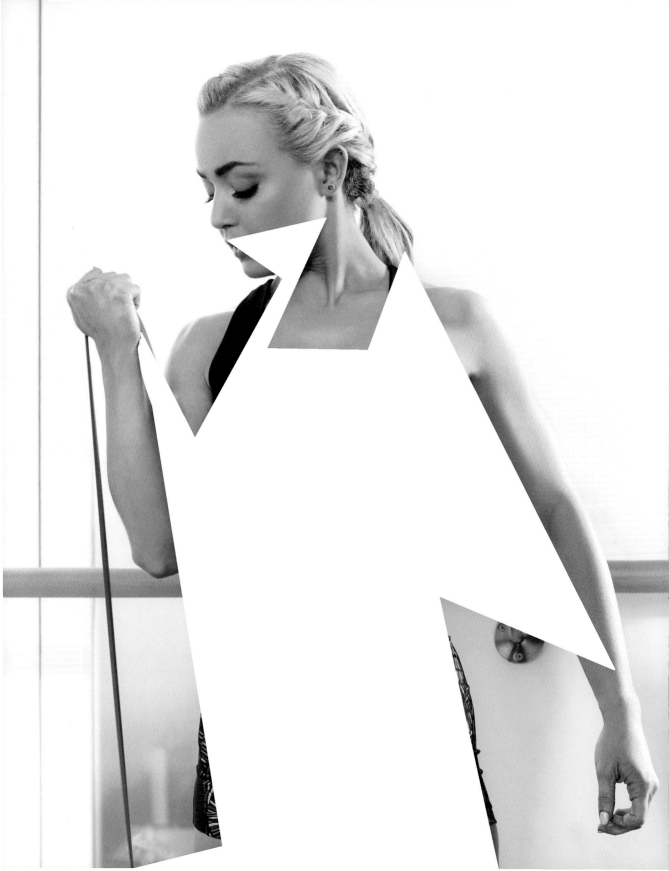

I know I have spoken about this before, so some of you will know I feel strongly about the issue of unqualified people posting information that hasn't been substantiated by a professional. It is so important with the increase in people sharing their 'knowledge' to be doubly sure where you are taking your information from. Anyone can post anything and call themselves experts, and it is so dangerous, in terms of both nutrition and exercise. Without knowing it you could be doing yourself real physical damage on both fronts, so the more you educate yourself, the more you can separate fact from fiction and stay safe. We only have to scroll down our social-media feeds to see how many people are promoting a certain way of life, or endorsing certain products, and to see that the fitness industry is groaning with people to follow and products to buy – all of which can apparently guarantee us the 'magic' answer to what we want. But these 'answers' fail to address the fact that we all want and need different things, and no two bodies or minds are the same. I do think that there are some universal concepts that hold for us all – mainly that we all want to look as good as we can and, more importantly, feel as good as we can. We only get one body and we owe it to ourselves to do the best we can for it and to it.

My first book brought together food and fitness, and detailed how I got started on the right path – and stayed on track. My second book was dedicated to nutrition and how you can nourish and fuel your body to make sure it achieves its maximum potential. For me now, food and exercise are at the centre of my life – I eat as well as I can and I spend my day training clients to push themselves as much as they can. I try and give as much context as I can with my clients, but simply reading around the subject, for example on topics such as mobility, recovery or weight-training, can allow you to build a much broader knowledge of exercise, empowering you to make much more educated decisions when it comes to deciding how to approach your own training.

HERE ARE A FEW OF MY FAVOURITE BOOKS AND PODCASTS TO GIVE YOU SOMEWHERE TO START WITH YOUR OWN READING AND RESEARCH:

Becoming a Supple Leopard – Dr Kelly Starrett
Strength Training Anatomy – Frederic Delavier
Weight Training for Dummies – Liz Neporent, Suzanne Schlosberg and Shirley J. Archer
Ben Coomber podcast
The Performance podcast
Sigma Nutrition podcast
The Nutrition Diva podcast
Real Nutrition Radio

CLIENT TESTIMONIAL: JENNY

I have been training with Alice for a number of months now, and I can honestly say that I have loved every session with her more than the last. Alice is a passionate young lady who aims to explain every decision within our session, instead of just throwing exercises at me. She, on numerous occasions, has come into our session excited after having read research and then applied it to our training, and it's inspiring to work with someone who cares so much about her work. I have gained not only strength, but also so much confidence since training with Alice, and long may it continue!

MAINTAINING PROGRESS

TRACK YOUR PROGRESSION

All of the workouts within this book are designed in a way that makes it easy to track your progression week on week. With any training programme it is important to keep note of what you achieve within each session so that you can see your fitness progress.

KNOW WHEN TO REST

When it comes to exercising, it is so important to not overlook your body's need to rest and recover between sessions. Failing to take this into account can result in your body 'burning out', which can, of course, cause complete lack of motivation. For those who set purely short-term goals, it can seem sustainable to train multiple times a week and almost enter into a mind-over-matter mindset with muscle soreness and tiredness.

With this book the aim is to maintain motivation and activity levels year round, and for this reason adequate rest should absolutely be incorporated into your training routine to allow for consistent energy levels and the ability to get the most out of each session. We have all gone through that phase of joining a gym and going every day in an attempt to get value for money and prove we are committed, but this kind of pattern is not sustainable and that is why people don't keep it up. You need to be realistic from the very start and only set goals you can achieve in the first instance. So if you work shifts, say to yourself that you will work out for 40 minutes three times a week as a minimum input. It is all about starting off on the right foot and implementing something that you can stick to – anything extra is a bonus!

PRACTISE SELF-LOVE

This is one of my favourite things to discuss. When I began my journey, if someone had told me about 'self-love' I would have laughed it off as a hippie concept that really had no place in my story, but I can honestly say that it has been one of the best lessons I've ever learned, and something I now encourage all of my clients to work on.

I have recently spent time looking at more holistic approaches to wellness, and uncovering the benefits of making small changes to my lifestyle, which have made a big difference. These are little things that can be as simple as taking time away from social media, slowing your thoughts and taking a little YOU time in which you can reflect and achieve better clarity of thought.

I often find this requires me to do things like putting my phone on flight mode, running a hot bath and lighting a candle to create an environment in which I feel I can fully switch off. This isn't just me getting in touch with my spiritual side; multiple studies have revealed a correlation between elevated cortisol or stress levels and a decrease in many aspects of both health and happiness. For this reason it's so important to not necessarily do what I do, but to find your calm, and a space in which you feel you can properly switch off from the stresses of day-to-day life.

There is no one method of practising self-love, nor is there one rule book or magic formula to help you achieve it, but in my experience the most successful journeys begin with self-love and self-acceptance. Aesthetic goals such as dropping a dress size or wanting to shift stubborn body fat, in my opinion, only last so long before you can become disheartened with your progress. This in turn can put a negative spin on what should be a positive period of self-discovery and growth. We all have our body hang-ups, no matter what age, shape or size, and the first thing I began doing was drawing my focus away from the things I didn't like and putting a positive spin on the things I did like about myself. I had a long-standing cycle of negativity to break, and it felt overwhelming at the time.

With every new client I pose the question to them, 'What can I do for you?' and 99 per cent of the time I am met with the response, 'I'd like to tone up my stomach' or 'I want to lose my bingo wings' or even 'I want a better bum.' While all these goals make total sense, often that's not the whole story. This is because, no matter how hard you work (and even as your body changes), there is every likelihood that you'll then find something else that you aren't happy with, and so the downward spiral of body dysmorphia continues. By bringing your focus away from your body hang-ups, and instead learning to love the skin you're in through self-love and self-acceptance, as kooky as it may sound, this will only help you to see each progression as a real milestone, rather than an opportunity to find more fault.

EXPAND YOUR EXERCISE VOCABULARY

It would be completely impossible to include every exercise I have in my arsenal within this book, and that would also make for a terrifyingly overwhelming read. This book is an excellent starting point for any exercise newbie, or source of inspiration for those with a little experience under their belt, but I am under no illusions that it is the 'be all and end all' of your training. There are so many great variations on exercises, different lifts to try and different HIIT (high-intensity interval training) combinations out there, and expanding your own personal exercise vocabulary enables you to have more flexibility and variation within your training, which will, in turn, help you to keep motivated and not get stuck in a rut. My advice is to keep it credible by taking inspiration and advice from those who are qualified in their field, such as personal trainers and other experts.

GOAL-SETTING

I have discussed and touched on goals prior to this, and here I will help you to create your own bespoke goals. At the start of any fitness plan, you need to assess exactly what it is you want to achieve, and perhaps choose a variety of aims encompassing both short- and long-term achievements that you wish to accomplish. With all of my clients, the most important message I want to give them during our first few sessions together is to aim to make their goals life-affirming and practical, and not just aesthetic.

Practical goals can be anything ranging from achieving your first deadlift to completing a bodyweight push-up to simply increasing your activity levels throughout the week. For instance, if you struggle to do something like a push-up, or you've never learned to properly squat before, I'd encourage you to see these as things to work towards, instead of aiming to shift that stubborn bit of body fat on your stomach.

These goals are far more measurable than just looking in the mirror and focusing on your perception of negative aspects of your physique. There is no detox tea, ab crunch or magic wand that is going to help you spot-reduce fat, so it's at this point that I urge you to look past aesthetics and try to see the bigger picture. Aligning your aims to be exercise-based will help you to keep focused without obsessing over bodily hang-ups, and instead bring attention to your training, which will, in turn, bring about physical improvements.

While learning to be a personal trainer I was told about the SMART principle, and was encouraged to use this with clients. It's something I have maintained and applied to my own training and that of my clients.

SMART STANDS FOR SPECIFIC, MEASURABLE, ACHIEVABLE, REALISTIC AND TIME-MANAGED

SPECIFIC: It's important to create specific goals that don't just include vague ambitions such as, 'I want to lose weight, and tone up.' Focus on what it is exactly that you want, write it down and be specific with each ambition.

MEASURABLE: By creating specific goals, such as achieving a full-body push-up or training three times a week, you are able to measure and track your progress. So this is an excellent way of monitoring progress, moving away from a number on the scales and instead basing your fitness progress on practical achievements.

ACHIEVABLE: While it's totally OK to be ambitious with your goals, sometimes if they are too far-fetched your finish line can seem a million miles away, leading to a loss of motivation when you are a long way from reaching it. With this in mind, it's always a good idea to have both short- and long-term goals so that you have varying levels of attainability with them. With your short-term goals, perhaps focus on things that are weekly to monthly, such as aiming to train three times a week, or prepping a packed lunch every weekday, while your long-term goals could be things like achieving a full pull-up or running a half-marathon.

REALISTIC: There are some things we just can't change about our bodies. I'd love to be a little taller, but sometimes we just need to accept the bodies we've been given and learn to love the skin we're in. With this in mind, it's important to be realistic about what is actually achievable and what we must accept we cannot change.

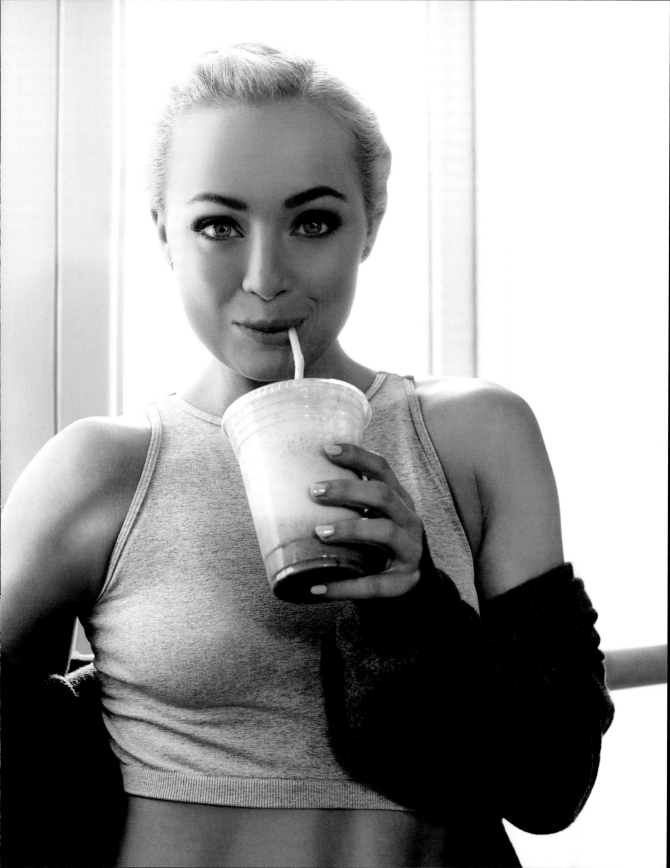

TIME-MANAGED: Having a goal with an open-ended completion date can cause you to lose motivation to achieve it, for the very reason that there is no definitive date set to reach it. By setting a time-frame such as three months to do 'x', you know how long you have to get to that point, and are then able to put a plan in place to achieve it.

So you now have the ability to develop your own personal goals. From here, try incorporating them into something that looks like the table opposite, where you can track and monitor how close you are to achieving what you've set out to do; from here, keep yourself accountable by sticking this up on a wall or on the fridge, and checking in each week to log your progression.

I thought it would be useful to include an example of how I structure my own goals, to encourage or help you to create your goals for your fitness journey. As shown opposite, I advise all of my clients, and urge all of you, to have a range of goals, from short-term weekly ones such as drinking more water to longer-term goals that will take a little more hard work and perseverance. These can be the silliest of things – and often simply just writing them down encourages us to actually do them, instead of them remaining as a thought in our heads – or they can be serious targets to spur motivation in all aspects of your life. Try writing this table out for yourself and filling it in with your aims, whether they are

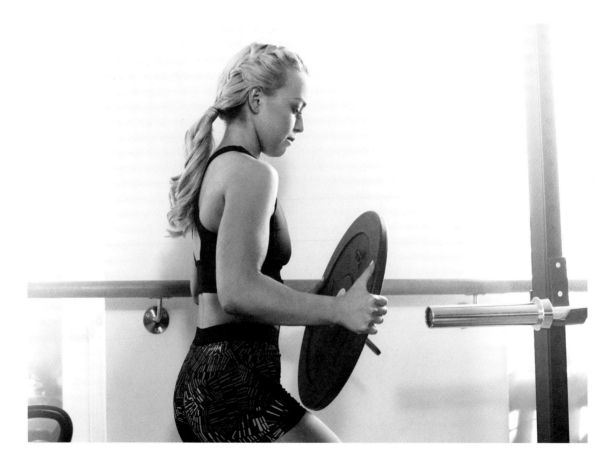

	THIS WEEK	THIS MONTH	THIS YEAR
FITNESS	Train four times this week.	Achieve a 70kg barbell squat.	Do a muscle-up.
FOOD	Prep lunches to take to work.	Don't scroll through phone while eating.	Experiment with more recipes, and make time for recipe testing.
LIFE	Don't use phone after 9pm.	Do more things outside the fitness bubble.	Become a UKSCA accredited coach.
DREAM GOALS			Achieve a BSc in Human Nutrition.

wildly ambitious (this is the place for dreaming, as I'll explain) or realistic and achievable. I actually do find that sticking my goal table up somewhere like on my bedroom wall helps to reinforce my determination to succeed in hitting these goals, instead of this piece of paper ending up buried under a heap at the bottom of a bedroom drawer.

I always include a dream section in my goal-planning, reserved for those seriously ambitious aspirations that might not necessarily be met, but are still worth writing down. As an example, a few months before I landed the cover of *Women's Health* magazine I wrote this as one of my absolute dream goals which I told myself would probably never happen but was exciting to even just write down – and look what happened! So, the moral of the story is, it's always worth aiming high as well

as keeping more realistic goals, as you never know which curve ball life may throw at you next!

It's also worth mentioning here that it is totally OK to *not* achieve goals, or to simply put them off until you are in the right mindset to achieve them. We never know what is around the corner in life, and sometimes when the going gets tough, the added pressure of striving to achieve set goals can often feel overwhelming. For this reason, it must be said that while goals are important in your fitness journey, also knowing when to modify them, or to put your health and happiness first, is of equal importance. Beating yourself up about not hitting set targets gets you nowhere, so be kind to yourself and know when to take a step back and try again when you're in a better position.

RECIPES TO FUEL YOUR FITNESS

While I have set out to equip you with as much training information as possible within this guide, I am first-hand proof that real physical change cannot occur without solid nutrition to support your training. When I first began my journey, I was at dance college, dancing up to six hours a day, and yet was gaining weight; a real testament to the saying, 'You can't out-train a bad diet.' For this reason I have included some specific recipes to help fuel and refuel you around your training. These recipes are designed with exercise in mind, and will focus on providing energy and aiding recovery so that you can really get the most out of your training.

Good nutrition is the key to everything, and I know from experience that you have to get that right before you can even think about anything else – a healthy body and a clear mind all start in the kitchen.

Eating around training is something I am often asked about, with so many people confused as to how they should actually fuel their workouts. I use the analogy with all of my clients that you wouldn't run a car without sufficient fuel in the tank, and if you did, you would find yourself coming to a standstill quite soon after you began. In addition, there is, in my opinion, such a thing as putting the wrong fuel in the tank, just as some people mistakenly, and often through no fault of their own, put diesel into a petrol-driven car, causing a whole host of problems. The same can happen within our bodies. Exercise requires us to increase our energy output, and when the exercise is intense we elevate the heart rate and switch to using anaerobic (without oxygen) energy substrates, in contrast to the aerobic energy system we function off day to day. This energy system functions, as stated in the name, without oxygen, and therefore instead runs off glucose, which is energy derived from our food. For this reason it is so important to ensure that the body has these energy stores in place, by fuelling up with sufficient nutrition to allow this process to take place. Not only will this ensure that you get the most out of your workout, it will also ensure that you're not eating into your body's reserve fuel supplies, leaving you feeling extremely fatigued by creating a huge energy deficit.

It's my mission to dispel any anxiety you may feel around food, and really take things back to basics in terms of simply getting a better understanding of the nutritional choices you can make around your workout without obsessing over this aspect of your training. To a certain extent, I often advise a little trial and error with your own nutrition surrounding training, to ensure you're not copying someone else who has totally different needs to you, and instead finding your own way of achieving optimal nutrition and working out how this makes you feel during training. I also must say that if you're really struggling I would advise seeing a qualified nutritionist to help you strike a good balance.

For those who are just needing a little inspiration, I've provided the following recipes, to hopefully simplify things for you and give you some ideas to incorporate into your pre- and post-workout nutrition. Each meal focuses on a good-quality source of protein, to help with the recovery of your muscles, and/or carbohydrates to fuel them with the glucose needed to energise or replenish glycogen stores, which will become depleted during and after your training. In my experience, many of my clients have varying times of the day that they train depending on their own lifestyles and schedules, and for this reason I've tried to incorporate recipes for those of you who train first thing, lunch-box ideas to fuel up for a lunch-time gym session, snack-style recipes for those who just need a quick energy boost pre-workout, and a few evening meal ideas to refuel after an evening gym session.

Pre- and post-workout nutrition is incredibly tailored to the individual, with different people responding differently to a whole number of variables, but I find a good rule is to try and eat around 30–60 minutes before training, and refuel within around the same window after you finish. If your training session is particularly intense or more of an endurance-style training that lasts a long time, you may also want or need to refuel during your session with something like a banana, for a quick burst of energy.

CREAMY BANANA AND DATE OVERNIGHT OATS

The perfect sweet way to kick off your day, rolled oats are a brilliant fuel to power you up pre-workout, with enough slow-releasing goodness to ensure your blood-sugar levels remain consistent throughout training. If you're enjoying this post-workout, try adding a scoop of whey or vegan protein to aid recovery.

SERVES 1

50g rolled oats

50g dates, pitted and chopped

1 ripe banana, peeled, ½ mashed, ½ sliced

250ml whole milk or unsweetened almond milk

½ tsp ground cinnamon

In a bowl, mix the oats, dates, mashed banana, milk and cinnamon until completely combined. Place the contents of the bowl into an airtight container and arrange the remaining banana on top, adding an extra sprinkling of cinnamon if desired. Cover and place in the fridge overnight, ready to enjoy the next morning.

ZESTY ORANGE AND LIME SMOOTHIE

Packed with protein and sweet sources of energy, this smoothie is easy to prepare and full of zesty flavour, to awaken your taste buds first thing in the morning!

SERVES 1

1 orange, peeled and sliced into segments

½ lime, juiced and zested

1 small handful of mint leaves, finely chopped

2 tbsp Greek yoghurt

5 ice cubes

Place all ingredients into a blender with 100ml water, blitz until smooth and serve.

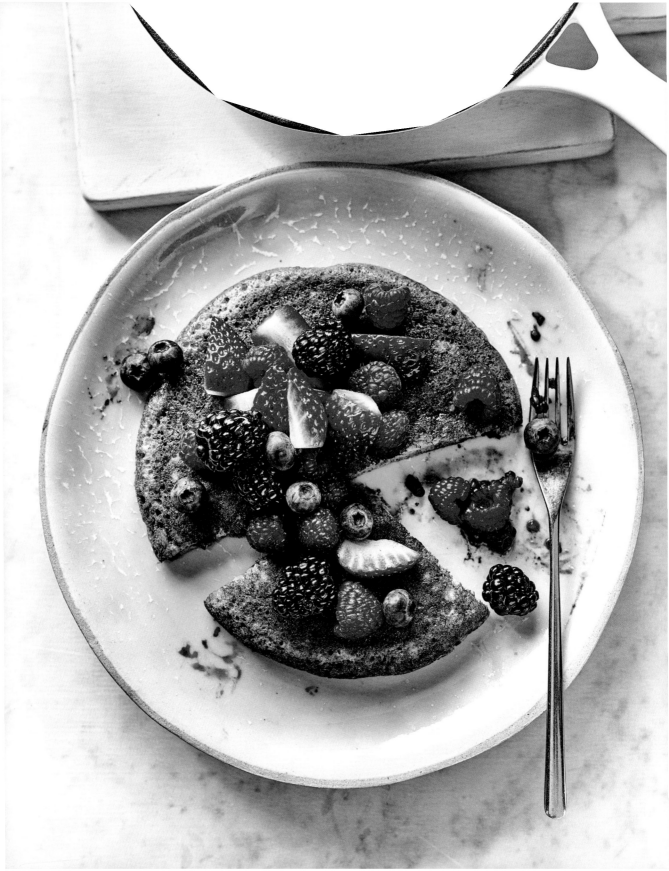

BREAKFAST
VERY BERRY SWEET OMELETTE

This is one of my favourite ways to start the day and is loaded with goodness to not only fuel a training session, but also ensure that you're taking on a wealth of antioxidants and good-quality protein.

SERVES 1

2 free-range eggs

½ ripe banana, peeled and mashed

½ tsp vanilla extract

½ tsp ground cinnamon

½ tsp unsalted butter

150g fresh mixed berries

Begin by separating the yolks from the egg whites. Whisk the egg whites in a bowl until they form soft peaks. In a separate bowl, beat the yolks until smooth with the mashed banana, vanilla and cinnamon. Combine the contents of both bowls.

Preheat the grill to high.

Heat the butter in a non-stick frying pan over a medium heat. Add the sweet omelette mixture and cook for a few minutes until set, then place under the hot grill until completely set and golden.

Serve topped with the fresh berries.

BREAKFAST
CARROT CAKE SMOOTHIE BOWL

A delicious twist on one of my favourite desserts, this smoothie bowl is a great combination of quick- and slow-releasing carbohydrates to provide energy for a workout, or replenish energy post-workout. Try adding a scoop of whey or vegan protein to aid recovery post-workout.

SERVES 1

1 carrot, peeled and grated

2 tbsp desiccated coconut

½ tsp ground cinnamon

¼ tsp ground mixed spice

1 frozen banana, peeled and chopped

2 tbsp rolled oats

250ml whole milk or unsweetened almond milk

Place all ingredients into a blender, blitz until smooth and serve.

SIMPLE CHEESE AND HERB OMELETTE

Simple doesn't equate to boring, and this omelette is loaded with flavour, a good-quality source of protein and healthy fats to aid recovery and keep you satiated throughout the morning.

SERVES 1

3 free-range eggs

½ tsp unsalted butter

50g Parmesan cheese, freshly grated

1 small handful of fresh basil leaves, finely chopped

sea salt and freshly ground black pepper

Beat the eggs in a bowl using a fork, then season well with salt and pepper.

Heat the butter in a non-stick frying pan over a medium heat. Add the eggs and sprinkle over the Parmesan and basil.

Once the base has set, fold the omelette in half and leave for around a minute, before serving.

PERFECTLY SIMPLE PROTEIN PANCAKES

Who doesn't love pancakes? These foolproof pancakes are a firm favourite of mine. Separating the egg white helps to increase their fluffiness.

SERVES 1

2 free-range eggs

1 ripe banana, peeled and mashed

1 scoop of whey or vegan protein

¼ tsp baking powder

½ tsp ground cinnamon

½ tsp coconut oil

150g of your favourite fruit, a dollop of yoghurt and toasted coconut flakes, to serve

Begin by separating the eggs. Beat the whites vigorously for a few minutes. In a separate bowl, beat the yolks until smooth, then combine both.

Add the banana, whey or vegan protein, baking powder and cinnamon and mix until fully combined.

Heat the coconut oil in a large non-stick frying pan. Pour a quarter of the pancake mixture into the pan and repeat until all the mixture is used up (you may have to do this in batches).

Once the pancakes begin to bubble on the top, gently flip over and cook for a further few moments, before serving.

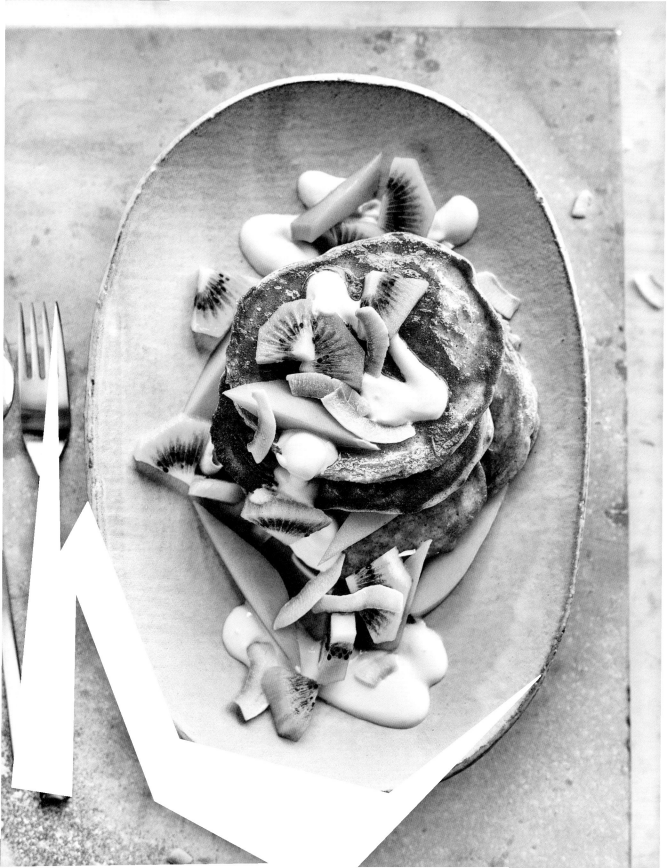

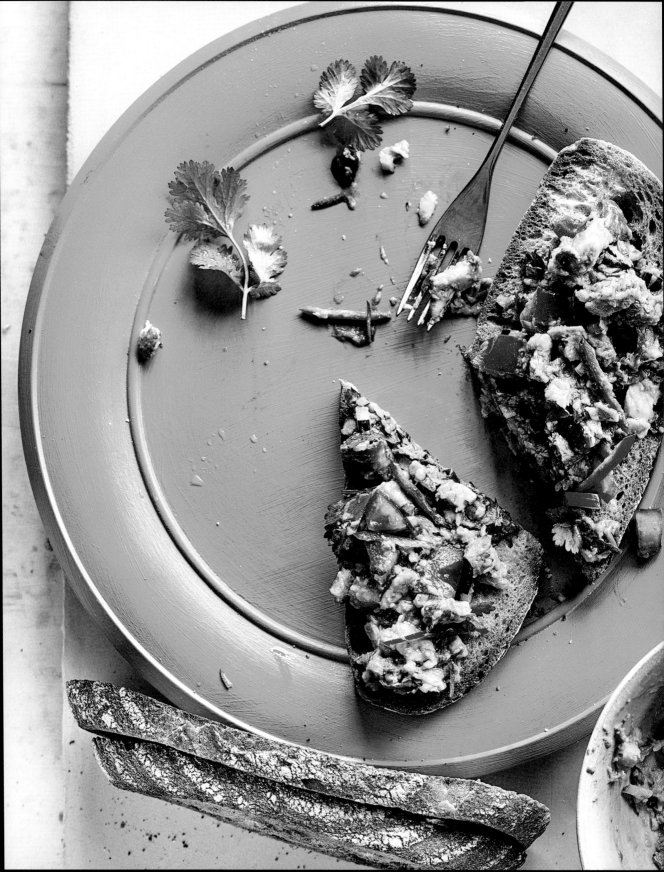

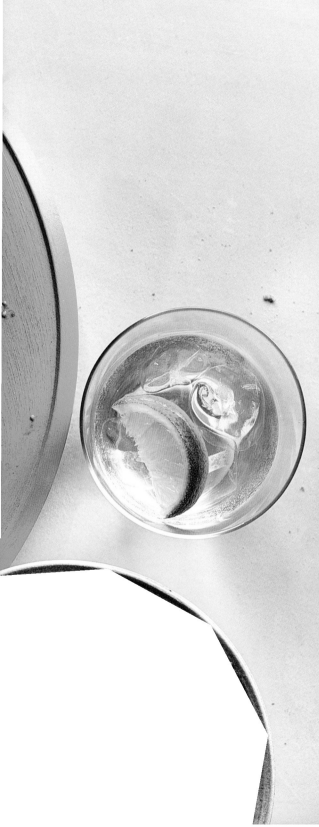

HOMEMADE GUACAMOLE ON TOAST

For those of you who fancy a more savoury start to the day, this simple combination never gets old. This breakfast provides you with a great source of healthy fats, fibre and a slow-releasing energy source!

SERVES 1

½ ripe avocado, peeled, halved and stoned

1 ripe tomato, chopped into chunks

½ lime, juiced

1 small handful of fresh coriander leaves, chopped

¼ red onion, peeled and finely chopped

¼ red chilli, deseeded and finely chopped

1–2 slices of toasted bread

sea salt and freshly ground black pepper

Place the avocado and tomato chunks into a bowl. Add the lime juice, coriander, red onion and chilli and mash together with a fork until completely combined. Season to taste and serve on freshly toasted bread.

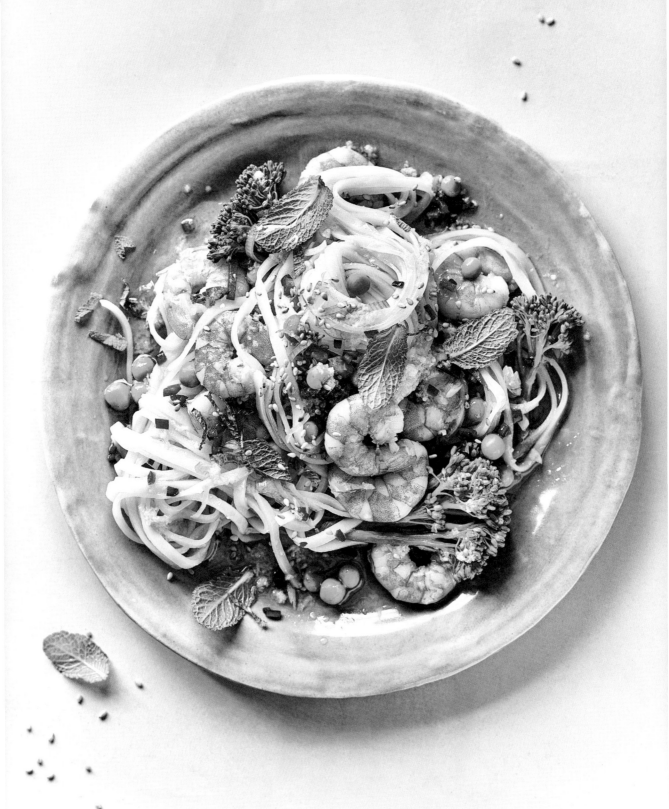

SESAME PRAWN NOODLE SALAD

I am a huge fan of prawns, and love the combination of spicy chilli and ginger to give this dish a kick!

SERVES 1

50g medium rice noodles

100g tenderstem broccoli

50g frozen peas

1 tsp sesame seeds

150g cooked prawns

1 spring onion, finely chopped

1 small handful of fresh mint leaves, chopped

sea salt and freshly ground black pepper

FOR THE DRESSING

1 tbsp extra virgin olive oil

½ tsp ginger, peeled and grated

1 small garlic clove, peeled and crushed

1 red chilli, deseeded and finely chopped

½ lime, juiced

Begin by cooking the noodles according to the packet instructions.

In a pan of boiling salted water, cook the broccoli and peas for 3–5 minutes until the peas are cooked and the broccoli is al dente. Drain.

Toast the sesame seeds in a dry pan over a medium heat for 1–2 minutes until lightly golden, then leave to cool. Meanwhile, combine all the dressing ingredients in a lidded jar and shake well.

Toss the noodles with the prawns, broccoli, peas, spring onion, mint and dressing. Sprinkle with the sesame seeds, season and place in a container.

TUNA, AVOCADO AND QUINOA LUNCH BOX

Simple and so refreshing, this zingy salad is the perfect meal prep to fuel you up for a lunchtime training session, or refuel afterwards. It's got a great source of protein, slow-releasing carbohydrates and healthy fats, creating an awesomely balanced lunch.

SERVES 1

1 tbsp pumpkin seeds

1 x 120g tin tuna, drained

125g pre-cooked quinoa

½ ripe avocado, peeled, halved and stoned

sea salt and freshly ground black pepper

FOR THE DRESSING

2 tbsp extra virgin olive oil

½ tsp sumac

½ tsp flaked sea salt

½ lemon, juiced

Begin by preparing the dressing: mix the olive oil, sumac, sea salt and lemon juice.

Preheat the grill to medium, lay the pumpkin seeds on a baking tray and toast under the hot grill for 4–5 minutes.

Meanwhile chop the avocado, mix with the tuna, cooked quinoa and season well. Finally drizzle over the dressing, top with the toasted seeds and place in a container.

LENTIL, SQUASH AND SPINACH DHAL

This dhal is the perfect cook-once, eat-twice dish that delivers protein, carbohydrates and a whole load of flavour. If you're wanting some extra protein, try adding some juicy grilled chicken thighs to the mix.

SERVES 1

½ tsp coconut oil

½ large onion, peeled and finely chopped

¼ vegetable stock cube

1 garlic clove, peeled and crushed

1 tsp finely grated ginger

1 small red chilli, deseeded and finely chopped

½ tsp turmeric

100g cherry tomatoes

150g butternut squash, peeled and diced

70g quick-cook lentils, rinsed and drained

100g baby spinach

sea salt and freshly ground black pepper

Heat the oil in a pan over a medium heat and cook the onion until softened, stirring occasionally. Dissolve the stock cube in 150ml boiling water and set aside. Add the garlic, ginger, chilli and turmeric to the onion and cook for 1 minute, stirring. Add the tomatoes and cook for a further minute, then add the squash, lentils and stock. Season with salt and pepper and bring to the boil.

Once boiling, reduce the heat and simmer for around 15 minutes. Stir through the spinach and cook for a further few minutes before serving.

SPICY CHICKEN, SUN-DRIED TOMATO AND AVOCADO WRAP

Who needs to buy lunch when you can make this from scratch at home in only a few simple steps? Full of flavour, this is a sure-fire way to make your colleagues jealous! Just grill the chicken until cooked through and leave to cool before assembling.

SERVES 1

½ lime, juiced

½ tsp dried chilli flakes

½ garlic clove, peeled and chopped

1 wholemeal wrap

½ ripe avocado, peeled and stoned

1 grilled chicken breast, sliced

3–4 sun-dried tomatoes, drained and sliced

1 small handful of fresh coriander leaves, roughly chopped

Begin by mixing the lime juice, chilli flakes and garlic until fully combined.

Next, take the wrap and squash the avocado, into the centre of the wrap, using a fork.

Add the sliced chicken and sun-dried tomatoes, then sprinkle over the coriander.

Finally, drizzle with the lime and chilli mixture, tightly fold the wrap, slice in half, before wrapping in foil or placing into a sealable container.

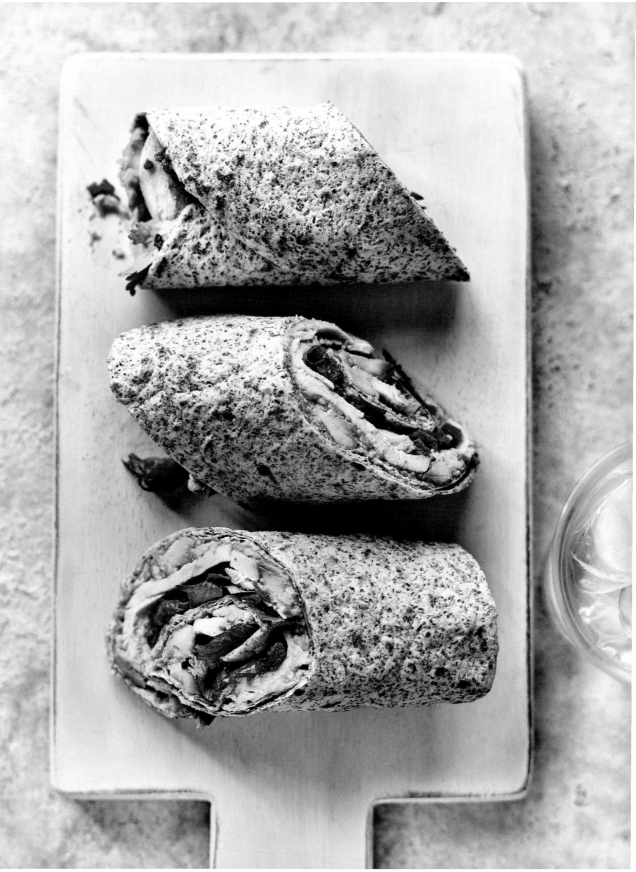

CRISPY SALMON AND CHORIZO WITH ROASTED RED ONION AND BUTTERNUT SQUASH

Loaded with healthy fats, protein and, most importantly, flavour, this dish is a firm favourite either pre- or post-workout, and will ensure you're fuelling your fitness right!

SERVES 1

1 tbsp coconut oil

150g butternut squash, peeled and cut into wedges

½ red onion, peeled and cut into wedges

a couple of sprigs of fresh rosemary

½ tsp chilli flakes

4 small slices of chorizo

1 salmon fillet

sea salt and freshly ground black pepper

Preheat the oven to 180°C/350°F/Gas Mark 4.

Put the coconut oil in a roasting dish and place in the oven until melted. Add the squash and onion wedges to the roasting dish, pick over the rosemary leaves and stir to coat in the oil. Season well with the chilli flakes and a pinch of salt and pepper, then cook in the hot oven for around 30 minutes.

After the squash has been cooking for 15 minutes, place a frying pan over a medium heat and add the chorizo for a few minutes until it starts to release oil. Add the salmon to the pan skin-side down and continue to cook for 4–6 minutes, then flip and cook for another 2 minutes or until cooked through.

Once cooked, remove from the heat and leave to cool.

Remove the squash and onion from the oven and transfer to a plastic container. Once cooled, add the salmon and chorizo, flaking the fish as you go.

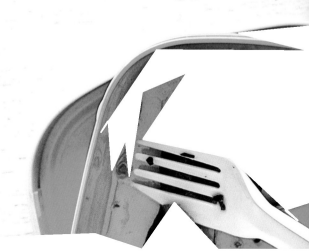

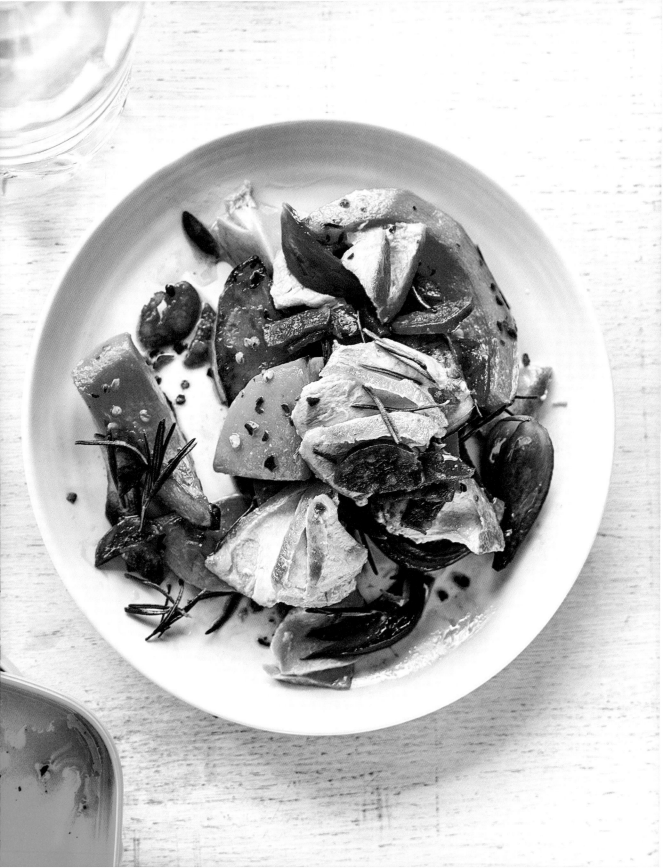

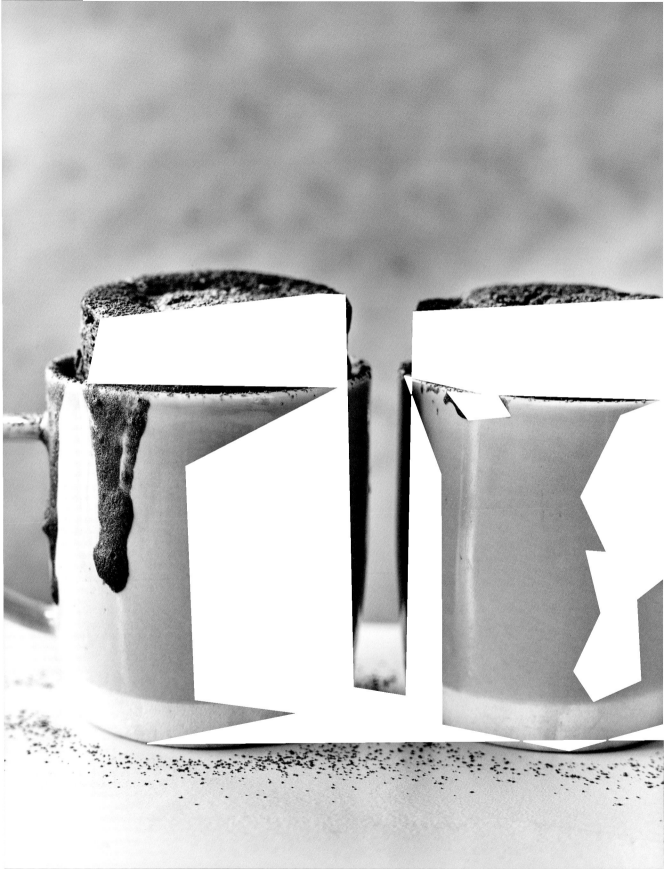

GOOEY BANANA, DATE AND CHOCOLATE MUG CAKE

POST-WORKOUT PROTEIN PUNCH

Cake just got better – this mug cake is the ideal fuel to see you through a sweaty workout. Try adding different dried fruit or nuts to find your perfect combination.

This recipe couldn't be simpler and is providing everything you need to refuel post-workout. With a good source of both protein and carbohydrates, this will ensure you don't experience a post-workout energy crash!

SERVES 1

2 tbsp self-raising flour

1 tbsp cacao powder

1 free-range egg

1 tbsp mashed banana

2 tbsp unsweetened almond milk

a few drops of vanilla extract

2 tbsp unsalted butter, melted

1 small handful of dates, pitted and chopped

SERVES 1

250ml unsweetened almond milk

1 scoop of whey or vegan protein

30g rolled oats

3–4 ice cubes

Place all the ingredients into a blender and blitz until smooth.

Begin by mixing the flour and cacao powder together in a bowl.

Next, crack in the egg, add the mashed banana, unsweetened almond milk, vanilla extract, melted butter and chopped dates and stir until fully combined.

Pour into a large mug and microwave for 3–4 minutes, or until fully risen.

REALLY EASY ENERGY BALLS

I love how easy these balls are to make. They're also brilliant for storing in the fridge or freezer to grab on the go, or take to work for a pre-workout snack.

MAKES 6

100g rolled oats

100g dates, pitted

100g sultanas

1 tbsp coconut oil, melted

1 tsp ground cinnamon

2–3 tbsp desiccated coconut

Place all the ingredients except the desiccated coconut into a food processor and blitz until smooth. Tip the mixture out and, using your hands, create small round balls. Roll in the desiccated coconut to cover. Place into the fridge for around 4 hours to set. Keep stored in a sealable container.

GREEK YOGHURT WITH EASY BERRY COMPOTE

This is a great snack to make if you've little time as it requires only a microwave to prep. As the seasons change, try incorporating different berries such as cranberries and blackberries to really make the most of the fruit on offer.

SERVES 1

50g blueberries

50g raspberries

½ tsp cinnamon

200g Greek yoghurt

1 tbsp pumpkin seeds

1 tbsp sunflower seeds

Begin by placing the blueberries and raspberries in a microwavable dish. Sprinkle with the cinnamon, place into a microwave and cook for around 1 minute before removing and mashing with a fork until smooth. If still lumpy, cook for a further 30 seconds and repeat.

Serve the Greek yoghurt topped with the warm berry compote and a sprinkling of the seeds.

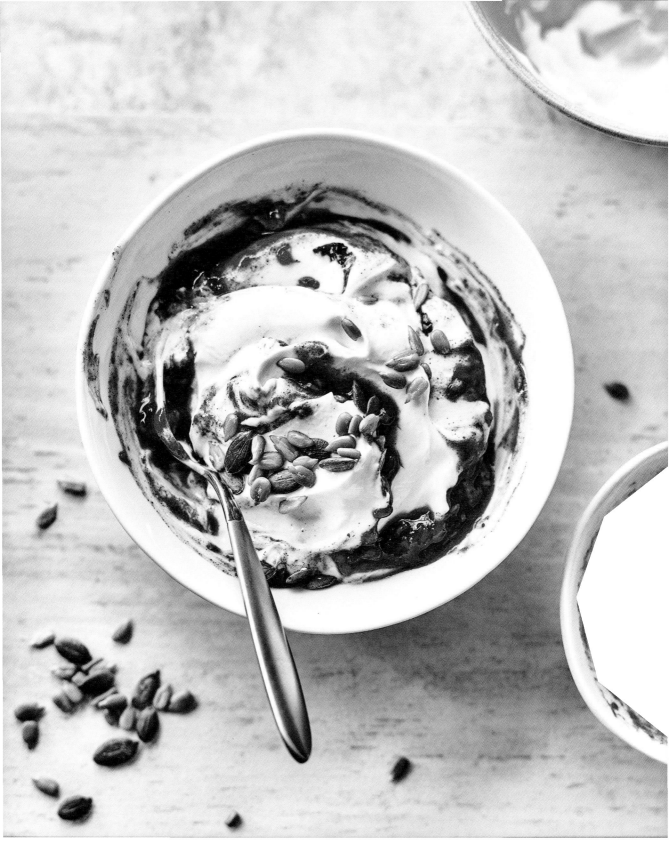

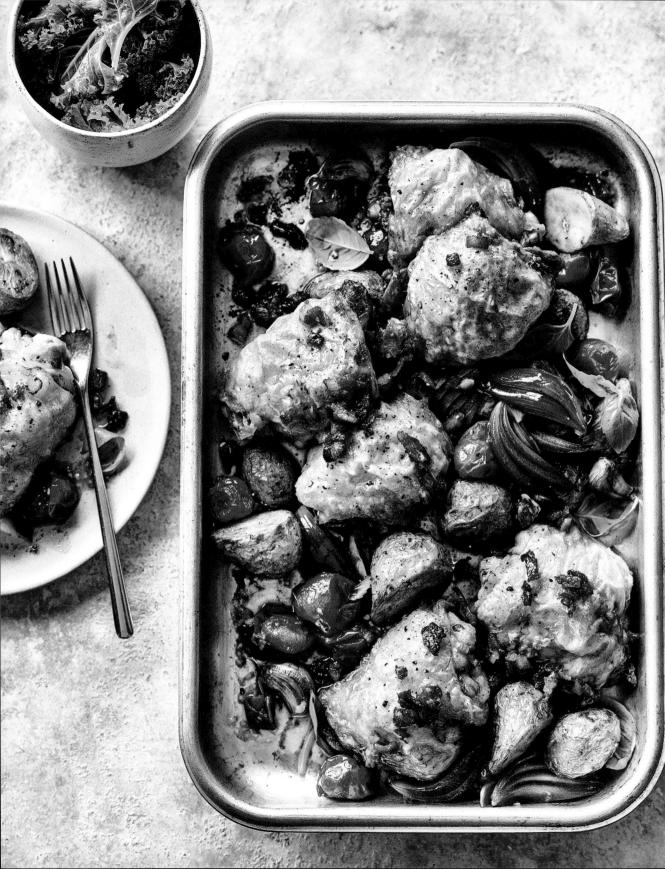

DINNER

CHICKEN AND BACON TRAYBAKE WITH NEW POTATOES

What could be simpler than a one-tray wonder after a busy day? It makes for excellent refuelling after an evening gym session! Pop the leftovers in a box for delicious lunching the next day, too.

SERVES 4

8 chicken thighs

200g ripe cherry tomatoes

1 red onion, peeled and cut into wedges

10 new potatoes

3-4 garlic cloves, peeled

1 handful of fresh basil leaves

3 tbsp olive oil

6 rashers of bacon, finely chopped

sea salt and freshly ground black pepper

Preheat the oven to 180°C/350°F/Gas Mark 4.

Place the chicken thighs, tomatoes, onion, potatoes, garlic and most of the basil in a large roasting dish. Drizzle with olive oil, season with salt and pepper and toss to coat.

Sit the chicken on top of the ingredients and cook in the hot oven for around 30 minutes.

After 30 minutes, sprinkle the bacon evenly across the dish, and then place back into the oven to cook for a further 15 minutes until the bacon is crispy and the chicken is cooked through.

Serve with the remaining basil and freshly steamed greens.

DINNER

CREAMY LENTIL, AVOCADO AND SALMON SALAD

Packed full of healthy fats, fibre and protein, this is a simple dinner that will ensure you're replenished and ready for a sound night's sleep!

SERVES 1

125g Puy lentils

1 salmon fillet

1–2 tbsp Greek yoghurt

½ avocado, peeled, halved and stoned, chopped into chunks

1 small handful of fresh mint leaves, finely chopped

1 small red chilli, deseeded and finely chopped

½ lemon, juiced

sea salt and freshly ground black pepper

Cook the lentils according to the packet instructions and leave to one side to cool.

Preheat the grill.

Place the salmon onto a baking tray, season well with salt and pepper and place under the hot grill for around 8–10 minutes, until cooked through.

Once slightly cooled, mix the lentils with the yoghurt, then stir through the avocado, fresh mint and chilli. Season well before squeezing over the lemon juice.

Finally, top with the grilled salmon.

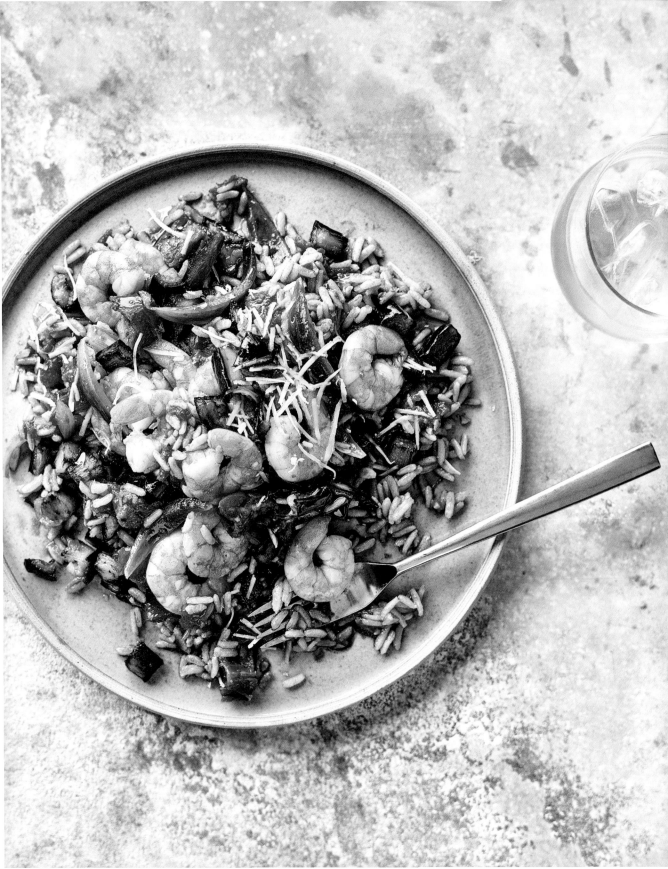

WARM KING PRAWN, WILD RICE, SUN-DRIED TOMATO AND AUBERGINE SALAD

Aubergine is my favourite veggie *du jour*. I love the simple combination of proteins, carbohydrates and fats in this dish. It's also the perfect meal to make once, eat twice, so you can enjoy it all over again the next day!

SERVES 2

2 tbsp olive oil

1 small red onion, peeled and cut into wedges

1 garlic clove, peeled and chopped

½ x 227g tin chopped tomatoes

125g wholegrain rice

1 aubergine, cut into chunks

150g cooked king prawns

5–6 drained sun-dried tomatoes, finely chopped

1 tbsp Parmesan cheese, freshly grated

sea salt and freshly ground black pepper

Preheat the oven to 200°C/400°F/Gas Mark 6.

Heat ½ tbsp of the olive oil in a pan over a medium heat and fry the onion until softened, stirring occasionally. Add the garlic and cook for a further minute.

Next, add the tinned tomatoes and around 250ml of boiling water and season well. Stir in the rice, bring to the boil, turn the heat down to low and simmer for 35 minutes or until the rice is tender.

Meanwhile, coat the aubergine in a little olive oil and lay on to a baking tray. Cook in the oven for around 10–15 minutes.

Stir the prawns, cooked aubergine and sun-dried tomatoes into the rice and leave to heat through for a further few minutes.

Serve sprinkled with Parmesan cheese.

EVENING DESSERT BOWL

I always like to finish my day with something sweet, and this dessert bowl is the perfect way to refuel after an evening gym session. Try making your own combinations to find the perfect flavours that work for you.

SERVES 1

1–2 tbsp mixed seeds

200g Greek yoghurt

½ tsp ground cinnamon

150g frozen raspberries (or other berries)

3 squares 80% dark chocolate, chopped

1 tbsp almond butter

Start by toasting the seeds in a dry pan over a medium heat for 1–2 minutes until golden, tossing often. Combine the yoghurt with the cinnamon.

Next top with the fruit, dark chocolate and toasted seeds, before drizzling over the nut butter.

EXERCISES

INTRODUCTION TO EXERCISE

So here we are. I hope the first chunk of this book has helped you to achieve enough motivation and inspiration to decide that there is no better time than now to begin your journey. While I can talk about my more holistic approach to exercise a lot, there is really one reason I feel so many of you have bought this book, and that is to hopefully let me help you to get fitter and stronger. Many within the fitness industry will lead you to believe that there are magic quick fixes. Or secrets that only few people know that will somehow fast-track you to achieve your goals, in my experience with my clients, no magic formula beats hard work and consistency for being able to see real change in your physique.

This is where the hard work comes in. With all of my clients I recommend at least eight weeks of training during which, with consistency, good diet and hard work, they will hopefully begin to see their body change and develop as they continue to apply themselves to their training. For this reason I also recommend that you don't look too short term with your goals to begin with, and instead allow at least eight weeks of consistent work before you then reflect on your journey and see how far you've come.

All the exercises included in this book are designed to be progressed with either reps or sets, tempo, or by adding resistance. Your aim should be to use these eight weeks to challenge yourself to achieve as much improvement within this time as possible. This is what we as personal trainers call a progressive overload, which in layman's terms means a gradual increase in volume, intensity, frequency or time, over a period of time, in order to achieve your target. This ensures you don't plateau in training, which can happen if you simply stick to the same number of repetitions, or lift the same weight over a period of time.

From here onwards, it's time to knuckle down and be prepared to put in what you want to get out of this book. I'm not asking for hours of exercise each day, nor am I telling you it's going to be an impossible task, but hopefully with the right mindset you will now be able to throw yourself into your chosen form of training, and start reaping the rewards.

So what are you waiting for? Time to kickstart your journey to feel-good fitness!

Within the next section you will find three different types of workouts: those that can be done from home, weighted and bodyweight short HIIT workouts, and gym-based workouts that require a well-stocked gym.

It has been my aim to make this book as accessible as possible, and therefore I know that it's not realistic to expect everyone to be able to afford a gym membership, or have time to hit the gym a few days a week. For this reason I've incorporated home workouts and short high-intensity workouts for beginners to grow in confidence, or those without access to lots of equipment in a gym. All the workouts included in this book should challenge you, and there is the ability with most exercises to progress or regress an exercise depending on your ability. As with anything in life, as a trainer I try and teach my clients that when it comes to training you only get out what you put in, and that means really trying to give 100 per cent to each training session in order to gain the results from your hard work.

It's important that you now focus on YOU. What type of exercise do you enjoy, and what is your starting ability? If you're a complete gym novice, I advise beginning with some of the HIIT or home workouts to familiarise yourself with various movements such as a squat. As the saying goes, 'Don't run before you can walk' … Weight-training can be a really effective training style if you know what you're doing, but for a complete beginner it has the potential to cause injury if exercises aren't executed properly. I always advise any lifting newbies to consult a trainer, even if just for a one-off session, as this will be of real benefit in the long term, building solid foundations to progress from. If you are more experienced, however, I recommend kickstarting your programme with a combination of gym workouts and HIIT workouts to really challenge you.

Don't worry if you're unsure how to structure your training – following this exercise section you will find a complete guide on how to personalise your fitness regime.

Time to get stuck in!

UNDERSTANDING THE BODY

In this book you'll find exercises that target various muscle groups within the body. To fully understand what muscles are working within each exercise, I felt it important to show you where they are all located, to help you achieve correct form and mind-to-muscle connection, in order to get the most out of each workout.

I personally felt it extremely beneficial to my own training to learn a little anatomy and understand my body better, so that I knew what each exercise was actually targeting, as I was then able to understand where the muscles were located within my body. I'm not asking you to become scientists, but even just a small glance over these diagrams can give you a better grasp of your body to help benefit your training.

The diagrams opposite show both the anterior (front of the body) and posterior (back of the body) muscles, and can be used as a reference as and when you need.

Within my own training I like to focus on training in upper and lower body splits, as well as throwing in the odd full-body workout – for example, training legs on one day, followed by training my upper body the following day. There are benefits to both styles of training.

When training in split body parts, some argue that you have more control over the targeted development of your physique. For example,

if there is a particular area you want to see improvement in, say the glutes, you can spend a little extra time focusing on that area in isolation. It can also allow for more effective recovery between your training sessions. Lifting weights isn't easy, and there is every likelihood that you may experience DOMS (see page 71) from a single session. By training in split muscle groups, a heavy leg day won't affect the next day's session if it is upper body, for example, and allows for more sufficient recovery. It also most importantly encourages us to focus on our weaker areas, which we can so often neglect in favour of training the parts of our bodies that we like training the most or are 'good' at training.

Having said this, full-body workouts can also be just as effective in helping you achieve your goals, which is why I try and incorporate a combination of the two into my own training split. In a full-body workout there are arguably a substantially larger amount of calories burned per workout in comparison with a split routine that is based upon individual muscle-group isolation. It also matters less if you miss a full-body workout, as it doesn't throw you out of a routine you may develop when using a more isolated body part training split. Finally, it can be great for beginners to get to grips with strength-training and build overall confidence in all major compound lifts. It is often the style of session I use with a lot of my clients who have little experience of weight-training.

Ultimately, the decision comes down to how often you are able to train and your own personal goals, and I hope this information helps you to determine what might be best for you.

ANTERIOR (FRONT OF BODY)

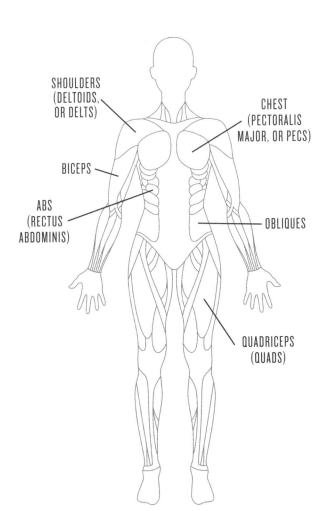

SHOULDERS (DELTOIDS, OR DELTS)

CHEST (PECTORALIS MAJOR, OR PECS)

BICEPS

ABS (RECTUS ABDOMINIS)

OBLIQUES

QUADRICEPS (QUADS)

POSTERIOR (BACK OF BODY)

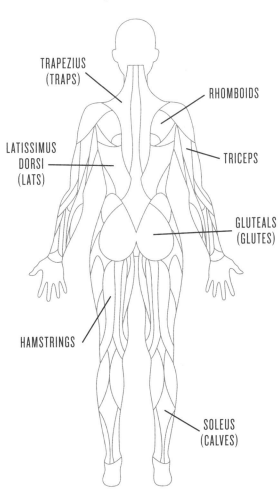

TRAPEZIUS (TRAPS)

RHOMBOIDS

LATISSIMUS DORSI (LATS)

TRICEPS

GLUTEALS (GLUTES)

HAMSTRINGS

SOLEUS (CALVES)

TRAIN SAFE

I've spoken about the importance of not overdoing it on the exercise front for many reasons, both physical and mental. The workouts in this section of the book vary in both technique and intensity and it's important to be aware of how your body, and in particular your heart, performs during exercise.

You often hear that exercise is about getting your heart rate up or getting your heart pumping, but what does that actually mean?

Different types of exercise will raise your heart rate by different intensities. For instance, very light cardiovascular exercise, such as walking, will raise your heart rate to 50–60% of your maximum heart rate whereas maximum-effort cardiovascular exercise, such as sprinting, will raise your heart rate much higher. Both types of exercises have their advantages, but it's important to monitor

how long you maintain exercising at a higher effort level. Below is a table that indicates how long you should sustain exercise at each effort level. Make sure you are training within the parameters below to keep your workouts safe.

An average resting heart rate for an adult is anywhere between 60 and 100 bpm (beats per minute). You can measure yours quite simply by feeling for your pulse on your wrist or neck, set a timer for 1 minute and count the number of times your heart beats within that minute.

TARGET ZONE	% OF MAX HR BPM RANGE	EXAMPLE DURATION
1 VERY LIGHT	50-60% 104-114 bpm	20–40 minutes
2 LIGHT	60-70% 114-133 bpm	40–80 minutes
3 MODERATE	70-80% 133-152 bpm	10–40 minutes
4 HARD	80-90% 152-171 bpm	2–10 minutes
5 MAXIMUM	90-100% 171-190 bpm	less than 5 minutes

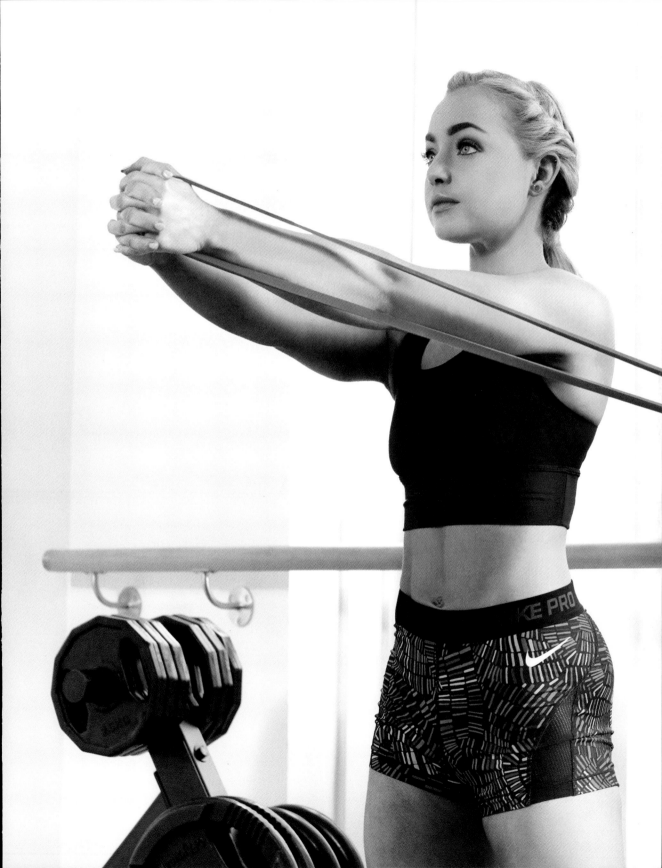

YOUR FITNESS DICTIONARY

The gym can be a daunting place, with all sorts of funny-looking equipment that can confuse even the most frequent of gym-goers. The same can be said for 'gym lingo'. Fitness professionals often assume that everyone is aware of some of the technical terminology used within the training environment, but I know I was often confused by a lot of the language used. For this reason I've tried to help you to get to grips with all of the terminology used within this book with this handy glossary, filled with all the slightly more obscure words and terms that you might not be familiar with!

ANTERIOR – the front of your body.

AEROBIC EXERCISE– 'with oxygen' describes a type of physical activity that increases the heart rate and promotes increased use of oxygen in order to improve overall body condition.

ANAEROBIC EXERCISE – 'without oxygen' describes any short-duration exercise that is powered by metabolic pathways that do not use oxygen but instead, for example, lactic acid or creatine phosphate, as with sprinting and heavy weightlifting.

BARBELL – a long metal bar to which discs of varying weights are attached at each end, used for weightlifting.

BILATERAL – using both sides of the body, e.g. both legs or both arms.

CARDIOVASCULAR – cardio exercise is any exercise that raises your heart rate.

CONCENTRIC – a concentric contraction is the shortening of the muscle during an exercise, thereby generating force.

CORE STABILITY – core-stability training targets the muscles deep within the stomach which connect to the spine, pelvis and shoulders. These assist in the maintenance of good posture and provide the foundation for all arm and leg movements.

DOMS – delayed-onset muscle soreness. This is the pain and stiffness felt in your muscles hours to days after exercising.

DUMBBELL – a short bar with a weight at each end.

ECCENTRIC – an eccentric contraction is the lengthening phase of the muscle during an exercise.

EXTERNAL ROTATION – external rotation (or lateral rotation) is rotation away from the centre of the body.

FATIGUE – muscle fatigue is the decline in ability of a muscle to generate force in a given exercise.

FORM – good form is conducting an exercise in a way that minimises the chances of injury for the person practising the movement. Good form also maximises the available strength and energy of the movement.

FULL EXTENSION – the point at which you return to your original starting position, for example in a squat, when you return to your standing position.

GLUTES – your bum!

HIIT – high-intensity interval training. This is a form of interval training, alternating between short periods of intense anaerobic exercise with less intense recovery or rest periods. It is a form of cardiovascular exercise.

INTENSITY – intensity is the amount of physical power that the body uses when performing an activity.

INTERNAL ROTATION – internal rotation (also known as medial rotation) is rotation towards the centre of the body.

KETTLEBELL – a large cast-iron ball-shaped weight with a single handle.

LATERAL – a movement to the side, e.g. a lateral lunge.

MUSCLE RECRUITMENT – the activation of a muscle.

PERIODISATION – the systematic planning of athletic or physical training. The aim is to reach the best possible performance at the right time for the given athlete, which involves progressive cycling of various aspects of a training programme during a specific period.

POSTERIOR – your bum!

POSTERIOR CHAIN – the whole of the back of your body from your calves up to the back of your neck.

RANGE OF MOTION – exercises that move each joint to the highest degree of motion of which each joint is normally capable.

REGRESSION – reducing or adapting an exercise to decrease difficulty.

RESISTANCE – this describes an exercise that causes the muscles to contract against external resistance to help increase strength and endurance.

RESISTANCE BAND – the elasticated bands that can be used to create resistance in a given exercise. They can be varying levels of strength or resistance, so can help you to regress or progress an exercise given the level of intensity.

SUPINE – lying face upwards.

TEMPO – the pace at which you move through a given exercise.

THORACIC SPINE – the middle part of your back.

UNILATERAL – using only one side of the body, e.g. a single-arm or single-leg exercise.

WARM-UPS, DYNAMIC STRETCHING, MUSCLE ACTIVATION AND COOL-DOWNS

THE IMPORTANCE OF WARMING UP

I often see people walk into the gym and enter into their training session completely cold, without even so much as a short warm-up. There are often multiple reasons for this: perhaps they're short of time, or are generally unaware of what to do pre-training to prepare their body for exercise, or they can't be bothered. Either way, in my opinion this only makes them more prone to injury, and also potentially leads to an inefficient workout, due to lack of muscle recruitment and muscle tightness, reducing the range of motion and mobility.

Warm-up exercises should always be specific to the sport involved, and I feel should promote mobility. They should exert sufficient effort to raise body temperature, and increase range of motion through the main planes of movement.

While I know that we don't all have hours to spend exercising, just a short warm-up can produce multiple benefits to your training session, and ties into my perception that exercise shouldn't be just about a calorie burn, or training to look a certain way, but optimising overall health. This means ensuring our bodies aren't just able to perform isolated movements within the gym environment, but to do these with the correct movement and posture, and without any impingements that can lead to injury.

In this section I've listed some of my favourite, most effective exercise-preparation movements and practices that I do before I train, to prepare my body for the session ahead. This is not a comprehensive list, but a handful of exercises that can help you to build and create your own warm-up repertoire personalised to your body and its unique requirements.

FOAM-ROLLING

Foam-rolling is something I do before my training to aid recovery, improve blood flow and help with the breaking down of muscle fascia in order to improve mobility and relieve any DOMS before I train. This can have benefits for improving your training session with increased mobility, and help to improve muscle recovery between your training sessions, too.

   With all of the following exercises it is important to apply necessary pressure to the required areas of your body, in preparation to train. Be mindful of your tempo, rolling slowly and with consistently applied pressure, rather than just rocking mindlessly up and down the roller. Use your breath to help with muscular release and gauge how effective foam-rolling can be for you, by judging its impact on your training. If you notice an improvement in your training, then continue, but equally, if you see little benefit, it is important to look at other reasons that may be hindering your training – perhaps a poor diet, inadequate sleep or dehydration.

FOAM-ROLLING
QUADS

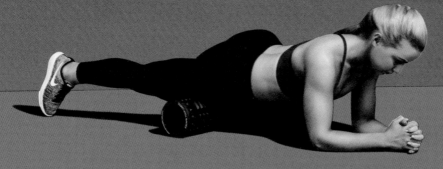

Place the foam roller under one quad at a time and roll gently back and forth.

FOAM-ROLLING
CALVES

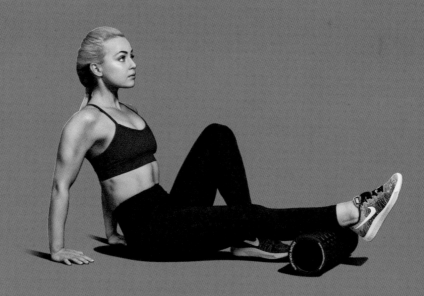

Place the foam roller under one calf at a time and roll gently back and forth.

FOAM-ROLLING
HAMSTRINGS

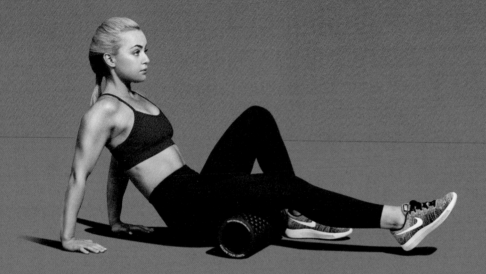

Place the foam roller under one hamstring at a time and roll gently back and forth.

FOAM-ROLLING
BACK

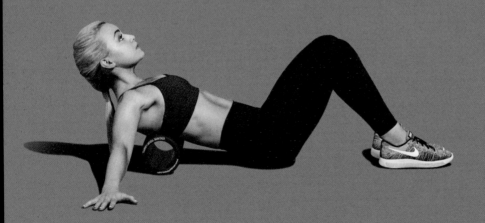

Place the foam roller under the back and roll gently back and forth.

FOAM-ROLLING
LATS

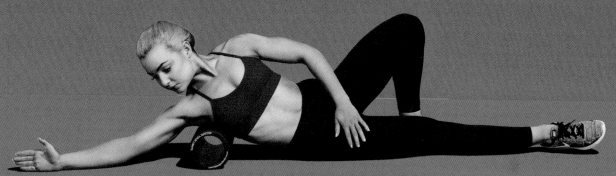

Place the foam roller under the lat and roll gently back and forth, repeat on the other side.

FOAM-ROLLING
GLUTES

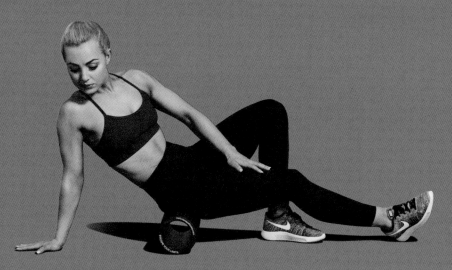

Place the foam roller under the glutes and roll gently back and forth, alternating sides.

WARM-UPS AND DYNAMIC STRETCHING

Once I've done my foam-rolling, I then progress to a small warm-up routine to raise body temperature, improve mobility and begin to prepare my body for training. Through my own clients, and in my own training, I have seen the benefits and performance improvements that can be demonstrated after completion of adequate warm-up activities. This is particularly true if you are new to training, as familiarising your body with different planes of movement, improving general suppleness and proprioception can dramatically improve all areas of your training.

DYNAMIC STRETCHING
LUMBAR TWISTS

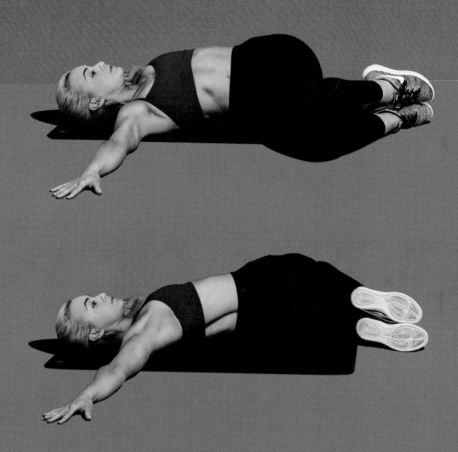

To mobilise the lumbar and thoracic spine. Lie on your back with your knees bent and your arms outstretched to either side of you. Gently lower both knees to one side and then repeat slowly to the other side.

DYNAMIC STRETCHING
LUNGES WITH THORACIC TWIST

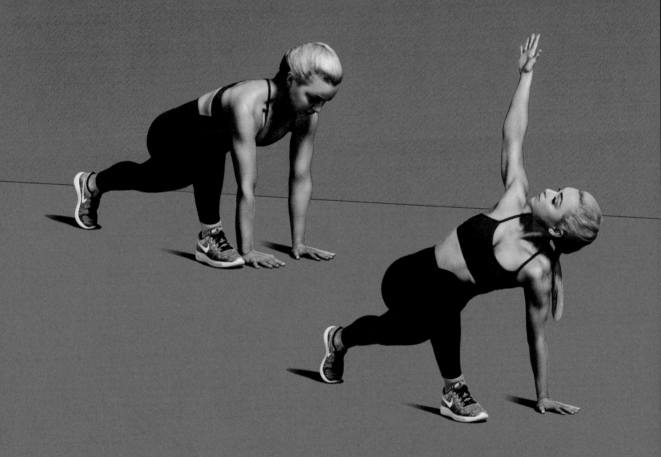

To further mobilise the spine and open up the hips, glutes and hip flexors. Begin in a plank position with arms outstretched and weight over the hands. Step one foot forward, to the outside of the hand on that side, and then open up the same hand and the forward foot, stretching towards the ceiling, feeling the twist through the upper back. Repeat on the opposite side.

DYNAMIC STRETCHING
SQUATS WITH HIP OPENER

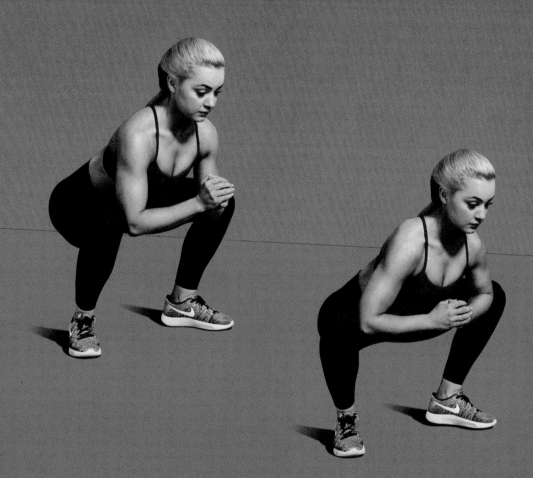

To open up the groin and glutes. Begin with feet slightly wider than hip-width apart and feet turned slightly out. Bend at the knees into a squat position and use your elbows to gently push out the insides of your knees. Hold for a few seconds before coming to full extension and then repeating.

DYNAMIC STRETCHING
ARM CIRCLES

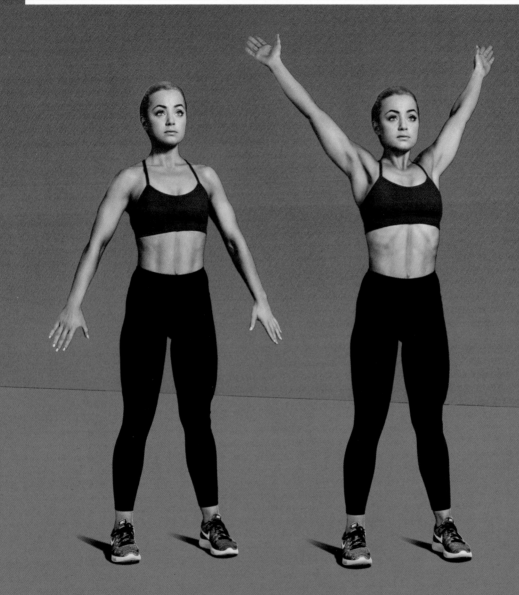

To open up through the chest and mobilise the shoulders. Simply straighten your arms by your side, and then swing forwards and backwards in a circling motion.

WORK OUT.

EAT WELL.

BE PATIENT.

YOUR BODY WILL REWARD YOU.

MUSCLE ACTIVATION

I am a huge fan of doing some form of muscle activation before I begin training, to hopefully increase and improve muscle recruitment and efficiency within my training. These will always be specific to my session, and for that reason I have divided the small handful of activation exercises into lower and upper body.

So many of us spend our days in a sedentary position at a desk, and therefore our energy output and overall muscle stimulation throughout the day can be minimal. This is why incorporating pre-exhaustive resistance exercises can help you to maximise your gym sessions by 'waking up' your muscles, in a sense, before you progress to the main phase of training.

MUSCLE ACTIVATION
CRAB WALKS

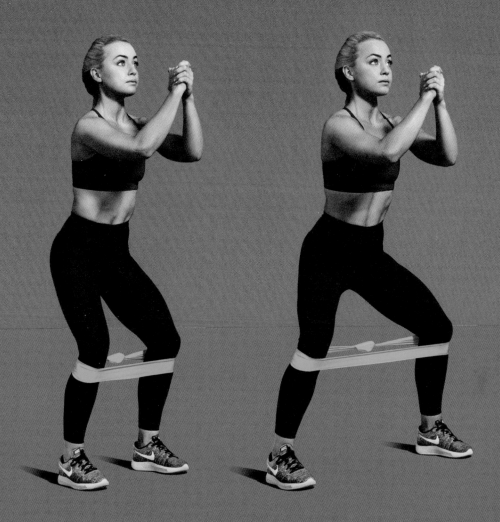

Place the resistance band just below the knee and bend slightly into a partial squat with both feet facing forwards at hip-width apart. Keep both feet facing forwards, step out to one side, bringing the other foot in to return to your original position. Continue for a few strides then repeat to the opposite side.

MUSCLE ACTIVATION
GLUTE BRIDGES

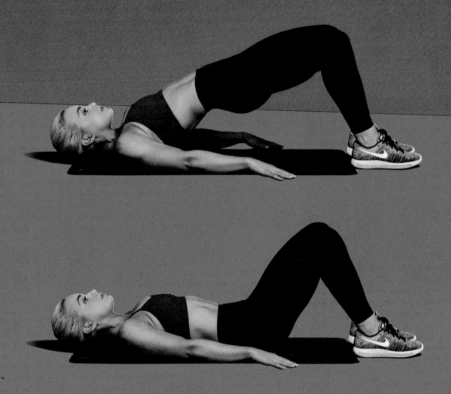

Lie on your back with your knees bent and your feet flat on the floor. Drive your hips up towards the ceiling, focusing on knees pushing away from the body, not hip height, to achieve maximum hamstring activation.

MUSCLE ACTIVATION
BODYWEIGHT SQUATS

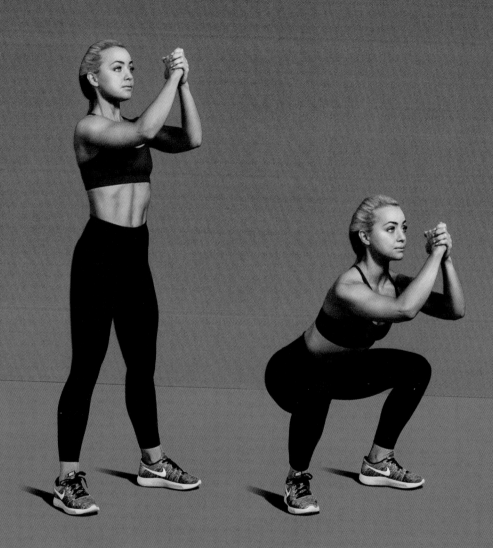

Begin with your feet wider than hip-width apart, with your toes pointing slightly out.
Keeping your chest up and core tight, squat down to a comfortable position without your
knees caving in, and then drive up to full extension.

MUSCLE ACTIVATION
MONSTER WALKS

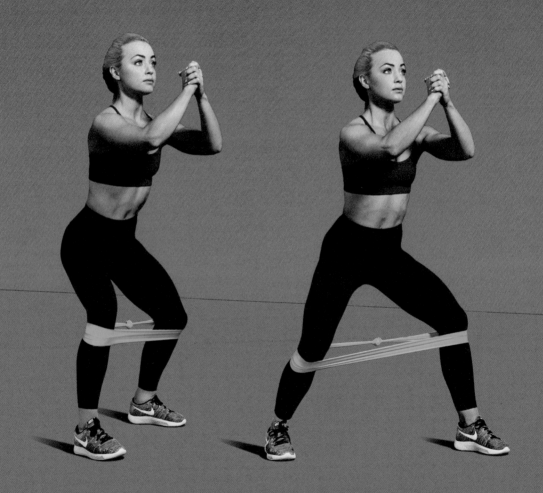

Place the resistance band just below the knees and place both feet under the hips. Step one foot diagonally forwards, keeping toes and knees still facing the same way, and then repeat, stepping the other foot diagonally out in the opposite direction.

MUSCLE ACTIVATION
GLUTE CIRCLES

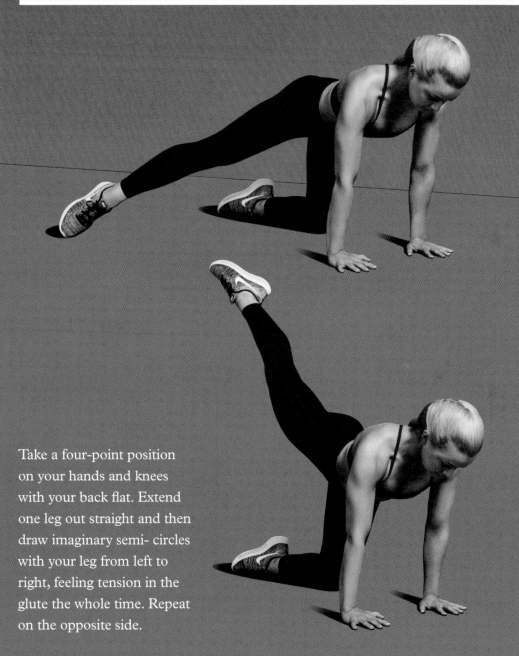

Take a four-point position
on your hands and knees
with your back flat. Extend
one leg out straight and then
draw imaginary semi- circles
with your leg from left to
right, feeling tension in the
glute the whole time. Repeat
on the opposite side.

MUSCLE ACTIVATION
BAND PULL-APARTS

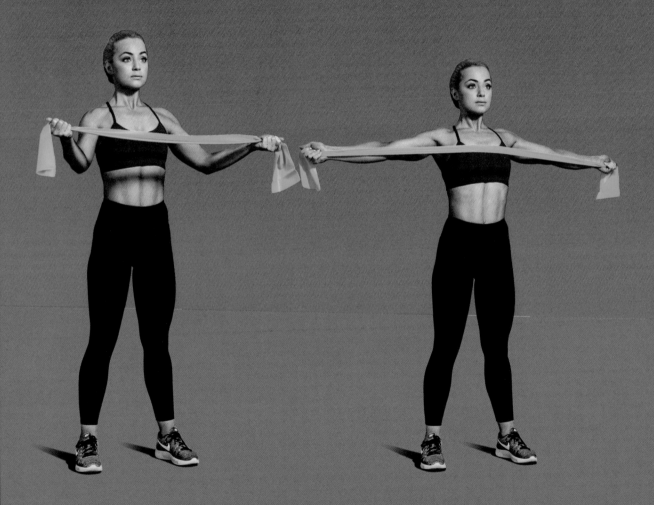

Holding your resistance band, take an underhand grip near the ends of the band and pull the band out and into the chest, feeling tension and activation through your back and lats.

MUSCLE ACTIVATION
BAND OVERHEAD CIRCLES

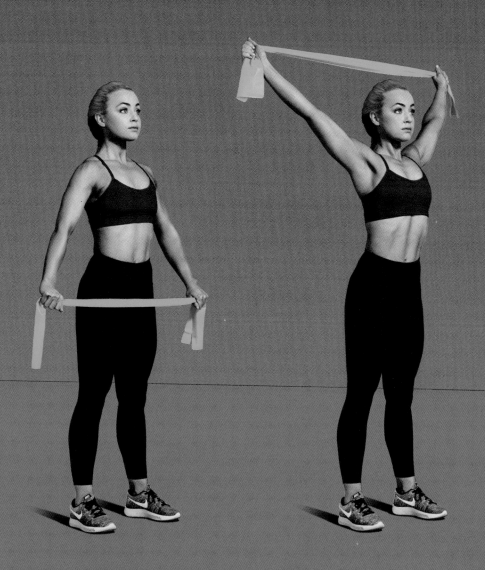

Holding your resistance band, take an overhand grip and slowly move the band in a circular motion over the head, feeling the mobilisation through the shoulder girdle.

COOL-DOWN STRETCHES

Once you have finished training you may find it useful to incorporate stretching while your body is warm, to help alleviate muscle soreness and improve mobility. Below I have listed some of my favourite and most beneficial stretches for you to use at the end of your sessions.

COOL-DOWN STRETCHES
HAMSTRING STRETCH

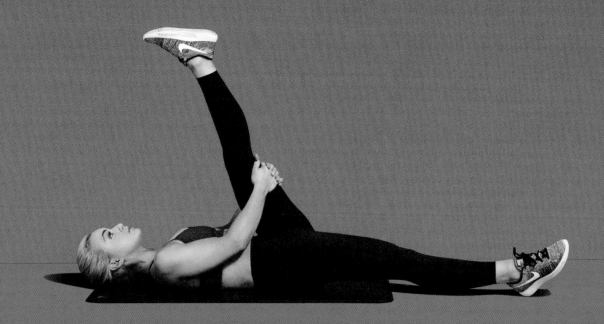

Lying on your back, straighten one leg and then draw the other leg into the body with both hands linked behind the leg just above the knee. Repeat on the other leg.

COOL-DOWN STRETCHES
QUAD STRETCH

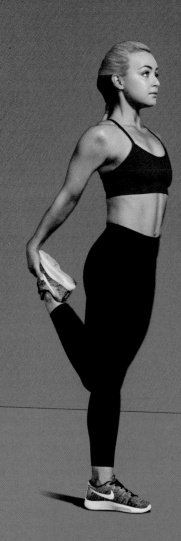

Standing on two feet, grab the foot of one leg and draw it into the glutes keeping your hips and pelvis in a neutral stance. Repeat on the opposite side.

COOL-DOWN STRETCHES
LUMBAR TWISTS

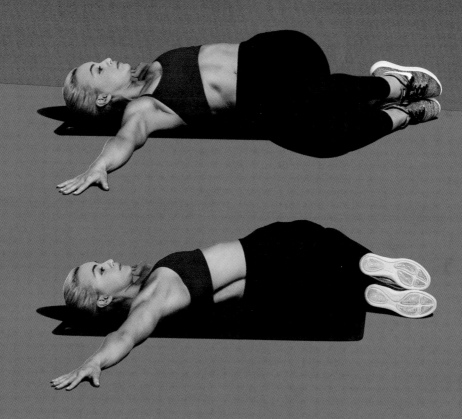

To mobilise the lumbar and thoracic spine. Lie on your back with your knees bent and your arms outstretched to either side of you. Gently lower both knees to one side, and then repeat slowly to the other side.

COOL-DOWN STRETCHES
IRON CROSS

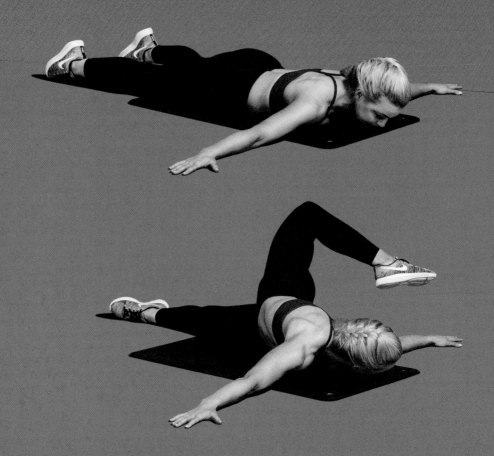

Lying on your front, with your hands outstretched to either side of you, reach one foot to touch the opposite hand, trying to maintain contact between your pelvis and the floor the whole time. Repeat on the other side.

COOL-DOWN STRETCHES
DOWNWARD DOG

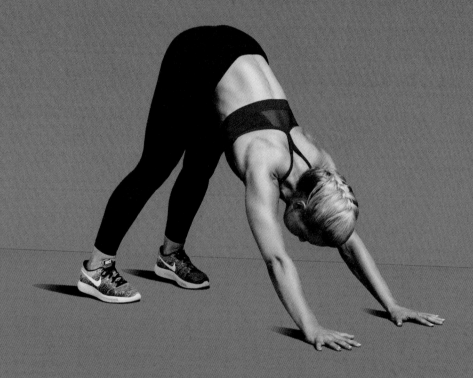

From standing, reach your hands to the floor, and walk them out so that you create a downwards V position. Aim to have as flat a back as possible and feel a gentle pull on the backs of the hamstrings.

COOL-DOWN STRETCHES
TRICEP STRETCH

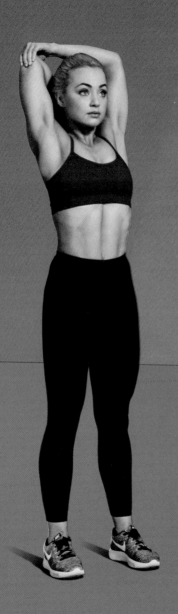

Reach one arm up above the head and bend at the elbow. Using the other arm, gently pull the arm to feel a stretch in the tricep. Repeat on the other side.

COOL-DOWN STRETCHES
GLUTE STRETCH

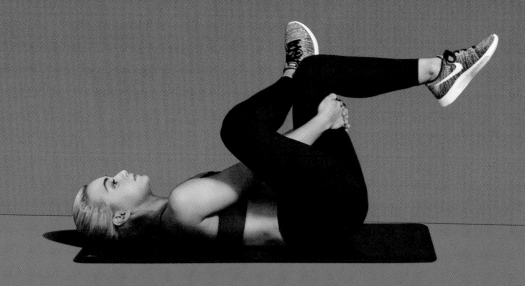

Lying on your back, bring your knees up to a 90 degree angle. Lace your hands behind one leg, and then cross the other leg in front of the leg you are holding, then gently pull your knee towards your chest. Repeat for the other leg.

HIIT WORKOUTS

HIIT workouts – high-intensity interval training – has recently had a surge in popularity. It is important to say that there is no right or wrong way to train, but HIIT can be an effective addition to your training if it is something you enjoy. I don't get as sweaty during my weight-training sessions as I do when I do more high-intensity cardiovascular style sessions like these, so I like to incorporate a combination of the two into my training regime.

HIIT training has been shown to improve aerobic and anaerobic fitness, reduce blood pressure and improve cardiovascular health. It is a great training style as it can be modified to people of all fitness levels and can be performed on all exercise modes such as cycling, running, swimming and so on. HIIT is also incredibly time efficient in giving you 'bang for your buck' with your training, and is therefore great for those who have busy schedules and little time to train. When you put in 15 minutes of hard work, particularly first thing in the morning, there is a real sense of achievement in knowing that you carry on burning fat long after your workout ends. The short, intense workouts also improve athletic capability as well as giving your metabolism a good kickstart.

Within this section I've tried to incorporate strength-based exercises within a high-intensity format to help build confidence in these moves for those who want to progress on to weight-training.

FULL-BODY HIIT (WITH DUMBBELLS)

This workout focuses on some of the main strength-based movements, from squats to rows, while also activating the core through full-body stimulus movements such as renegade rows and crunches. Adding dumbbells to this workout also increases the demands on the body and therefore increases the intensity and makes it more of a challenge – the more your heart rate goes up, the harder you will work.

Complete 45 seconds of each exercise, taking 15 seconds rest between each. Then repeat the whole circuit 3 to 4 times.

FULL-BODY HIIT (WITH DUMBBELLS)
SQUAT PRESS

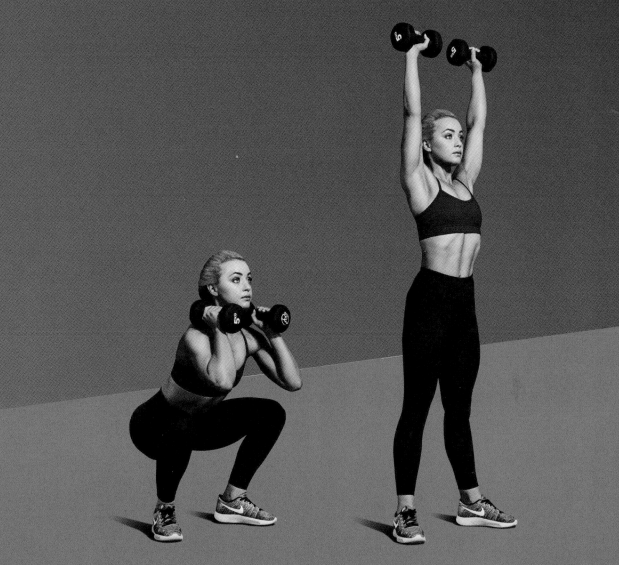

Begin with feet slightly wider than hip-width apart and slightly turned out. Place the dumbbells onto your shoulders with your arms bent. Keep your arms stable as you squat down, and as you drive up out of your squat, press your arms above your head.

FULL-BODY HIIT (WITH DUMBBELLS)
RENEGADE ROWS

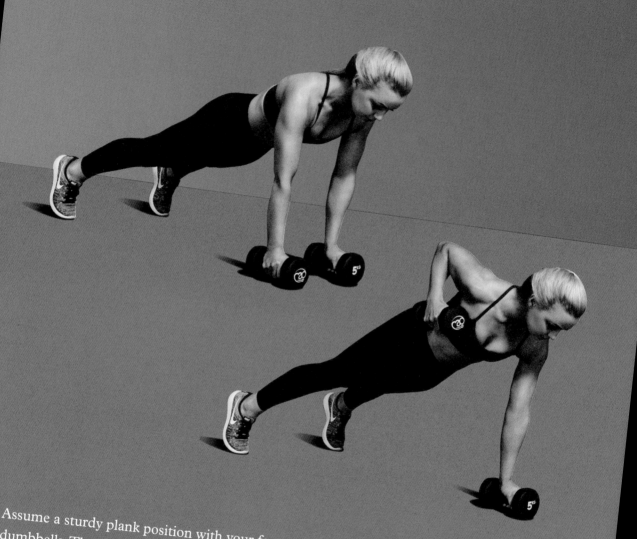

Assume a sturdy plank position with your feet set wide and your hands holding the dumbbells. Then draw one arm into the body, lifting the weight off the floor and keeping the elbow tight to the body. Set the hand back down and repeat on the other side.

FULL-BODY HIIT (WITH DUMBBELLS)
STEP-UPS

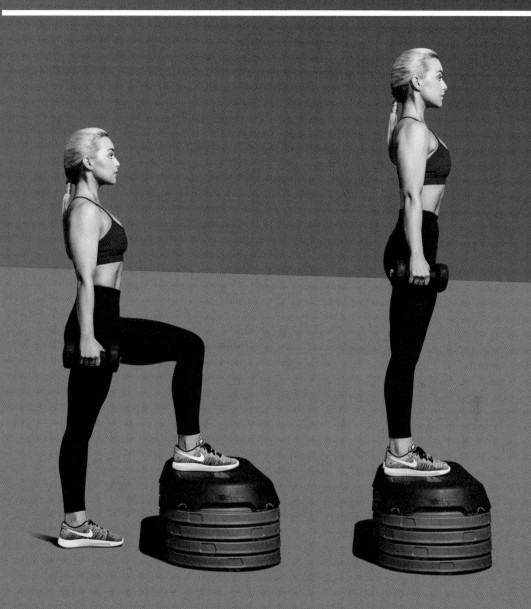

Step up with one leg onto a raised surface and step down with the opposite leg. Repeat, alternating the leg you step up with.

FULL-BODY HIIT (WITH DUMBBELLS)
SUPINE FLOOR PRESS

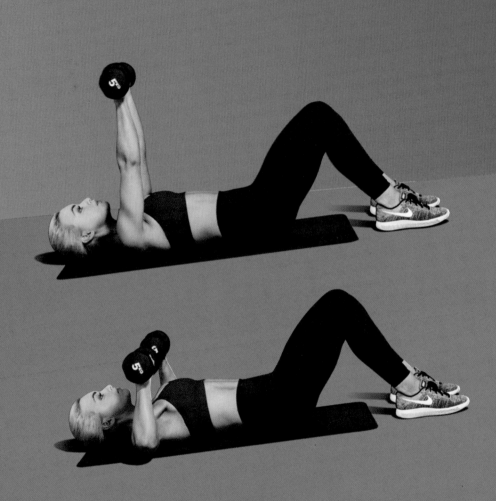

Lying flat on the floor, place your arms at right angles with the weights stable, then drive the arms up to full extension and slowly lower back down, and repeat.

FULL-BODY HIIT (WITH DUMBBELLS)
DUMBBELL ABDOMINAL CRUNCH

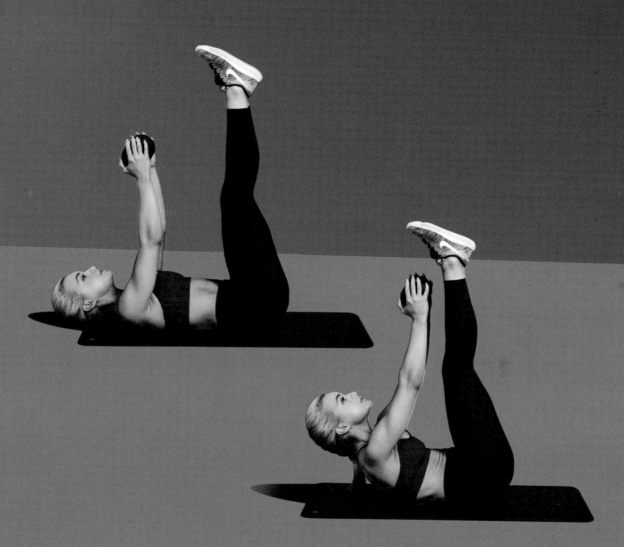

Lying on your back, raise your feet towards the ceiling. Holding one dumbbell with arms outstretched, bring the upper back off the floor, reaching the weight to the feet, and slowly lower back down.

FULL-BODY HIIT (WITH KETTLEBELL)

I love using kettlebells as part of my training as they are so versatile. This workout incorporates full-body exercises such as the clean and press, and windmills to maintain a high level of intensity on the whole body throughout. Any exercise where the weight is taken above the head also increases the stability demands on the body, meaning that the core has to work hard throughout, too.

Complete 45 seconds of each exercise, taking 15 seconds rest between each. Then repeat the whole circuit 3 to 4 times.

FULL-BODY HIIT (WITH KETTLEBELL)
GOBLET SQUATS

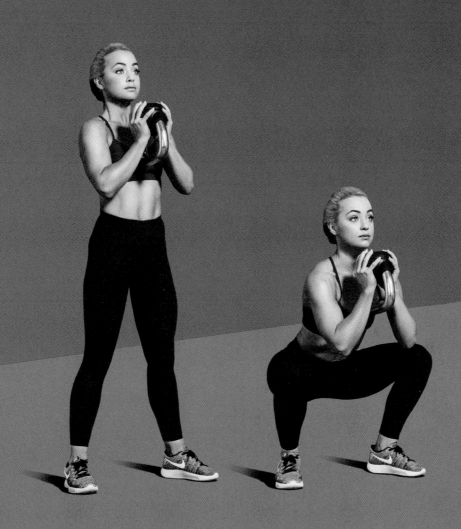

Holding the kettlebell in a cupped position, place your feet slightly wider than hip-width apart, keep your chest up and your core tight, and slowly squat down, ensuring your knees don't cave in. Then drive up to full extension and repeat.

FULL-BODY HIIT (WITH KETTLEBELL)
KETTLEBELL CLEAN AND PRESS

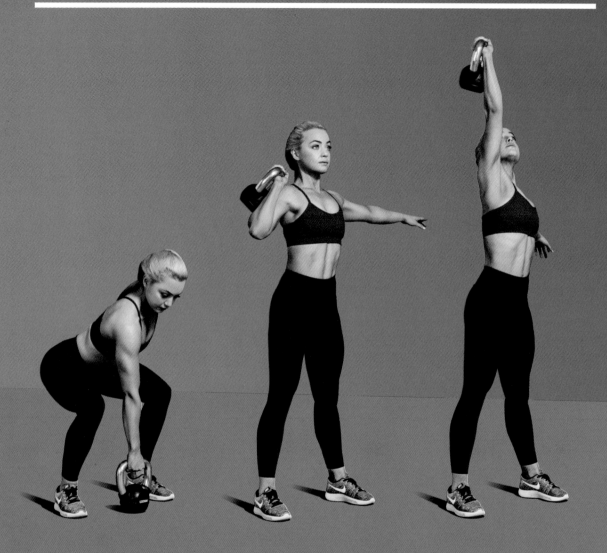

With the kettlebell in one hand, lower down keeping your chest upright. Touch the kettlebell to the floor. Next snatch the weight up so that it flips to behind your hand and keep your elbow tight to the body. Finally, press the weight above your head, lower down through the same movement and repeat on the other side.

REVERSE LUNGES WITH KETTLEBELL

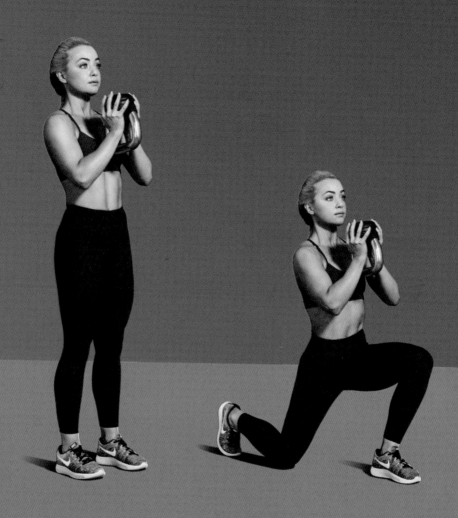

Holding the kettlebell in a cupped position, keep your weight evenly distributed between both legs as you step one leg back into a lunge position. Bring the leg back in and repeat with the opposite leg.

FULL-BODY HIIT (WITH KETTLEBELL)
KETTLEBELL SWINGS

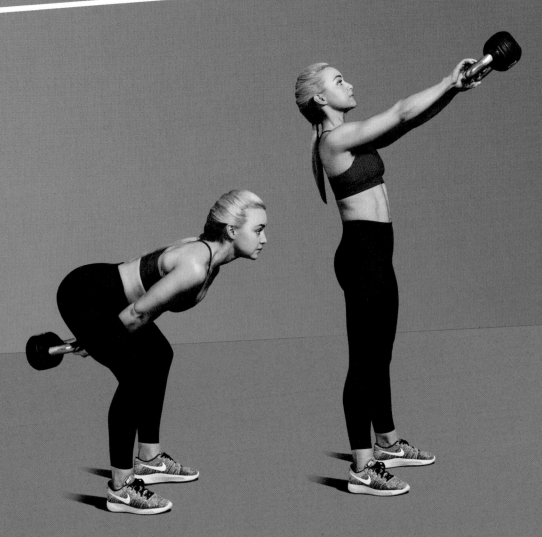

Standing upright and holding the weight in both hands, reach the kettlebell through your legs with as little bend in the knees as possible, keeping the chest upright. Drive your hips through and use the force to send the weight up in front of you, and repeat.

FULL-BODY HIIT (WITH KETTLEBELL)
KETTLEBELL WINDMILLS

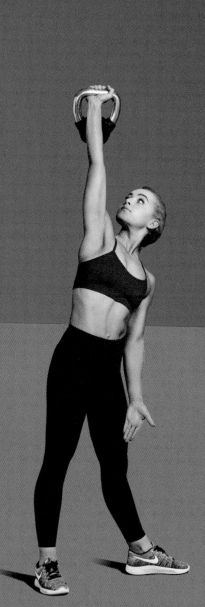
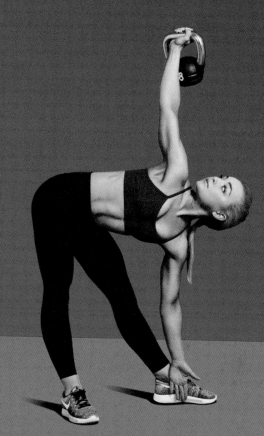

Standing upright and holding the weight with one hand, press the kettlebell above your head and turn the foot opposite to the hand above your head slightly out. Using your hand, track down the leg keeping your eyes on the weight the whole time, so you bend at the hip. Ensure you maintain stability in the shoulder and keep the arm straight and stable. Then drive back up to standing, and repeat.

LOWER-BODY HIIT

This circuit focuses on building strength through the legs and glutes. Aim to keep rest periods relatively short to maintain a high level of intensity. You should also try holding the weight close to the chest during exercises such as the reverse lunges, as they require abdominal stability to maintain correct posture, too.

Complete 45 seconds of each exercise, taking 15 seconds rest between each. Then repeat the whole circuit 3 to 4 times.

LOWER-BODY HIIT
GOBLET SQUATS

EITHER AS A BODYWEIGHT EXERCISE OR WITH KETTLEBELL

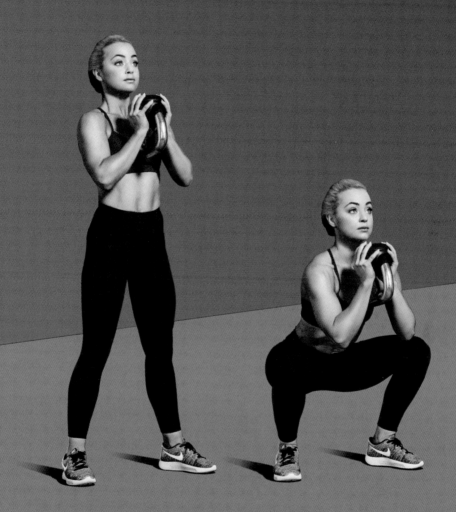

Hold the kettlebell, if using, in a cupped position or clasp the hands together if not. Place your feet slightly wider than hip-width apart, keep your chest up and your core tight. Slowly squat down, ensuring your knees don't cave in. Then drive up to full extension and repeat.

LOWER-BODY HIIT
REVERSE LUNGES

EITHER AS A BODYWEIGHT EXERCISE OR WITH A KETTLEBELL

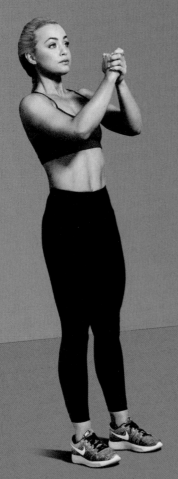
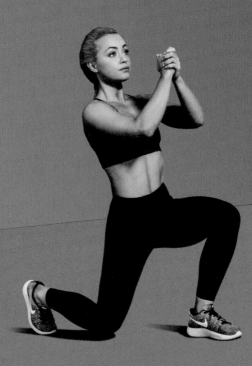

Stand in a neutral position with your feet underneath your hips. Holding the kettlebell in a cupped position, if using, or clasping the hands together if not, step one leg back into a lunge position, ensuring the weight is evenly distributed between your legs. Drive up to your original position and repeat with the other leg.

LOWER-BODY HIIT
STEP-UPS

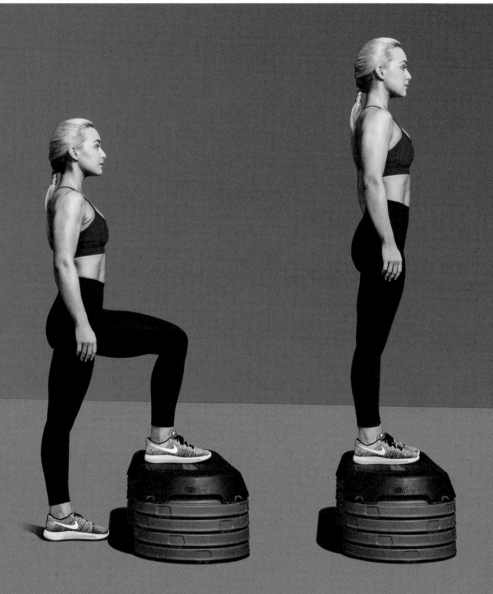

Step up with one leg onto a raised surface and step down with the opposite leg. Repeat, alternating the leg you step up with.

LOWER-BODY HIIT
RDLs

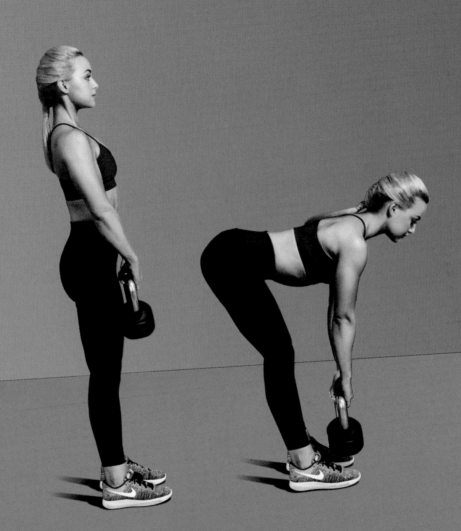

Standing upright and holding a kettlebell with both hands, hinge at the hips, keeping the knees slightly bent and the back completely flat until you feel a gentle pull on the hamstrings. Drive the hips through to bring you back to standing.

LOWER-BODY HIIT
KETTLEBELL SWINGS

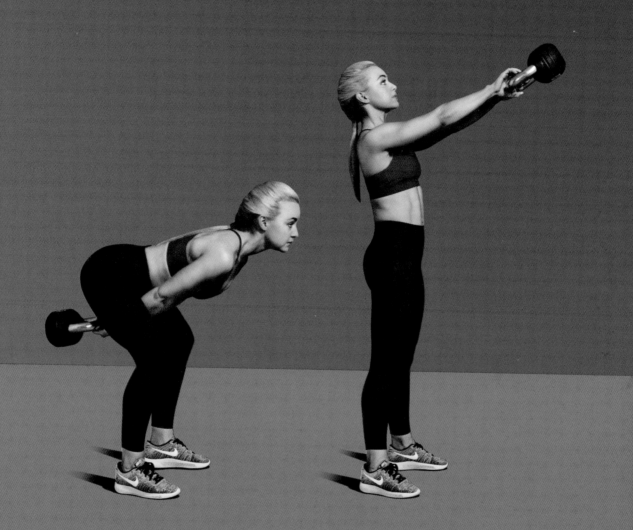

Standing upright and holding the weight in both hands, reach the kettlebell through your legs with as little bend in the knees as possible, keeping the chest upright. Drive your hips through and use the force to send the weight up in front of you, and repeat.

UPPER-BODY HIIT (WITH DUMBBELLS)

This upper-body circuit is a real combination of strength and high-intensity exercises, designed to build strength through the upper body with a combination of presses and rows, but also to increase the heart rate for increased caloric burn.

Complete 45 seconds of each exercise, taking 15 seconds rest between each. Then repeat the whole circuit 3 to 4 times.

UPPER-BODY HIIT (WITH DUMBBELLS)
OVERHEAD PRESS

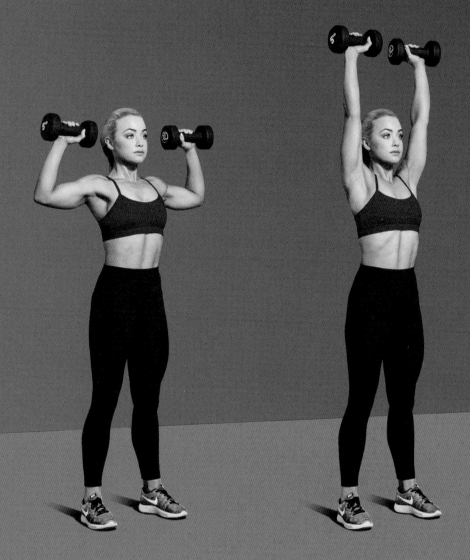

Take a solid stance with feet slightly wider than hip-width apart. Bring the weights to either side of your head with elbows in a right-angle position, and then drive the weights up above your head and slowly lower them back down.

UPPER-BODY HIIT (WITH DUMBBELLS)
RENEGADE ROWS

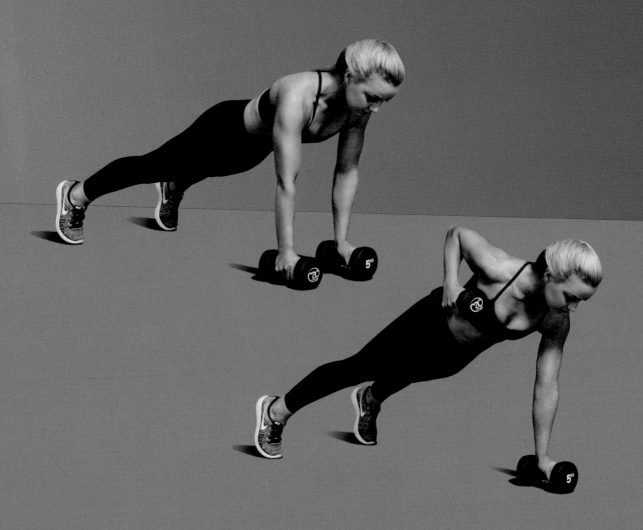

Assume a sturdy plank position with your feet set wide and your hands holding the dumbbells. Then draw one arm into the body, lifting the weight off the floor and keeping the elbow tight to the body. Set the hand back down and repeat on the other side.

UPPER-BODY HIIT (WITH DUMBBELLS)
SUPINE FLOOR PRESS

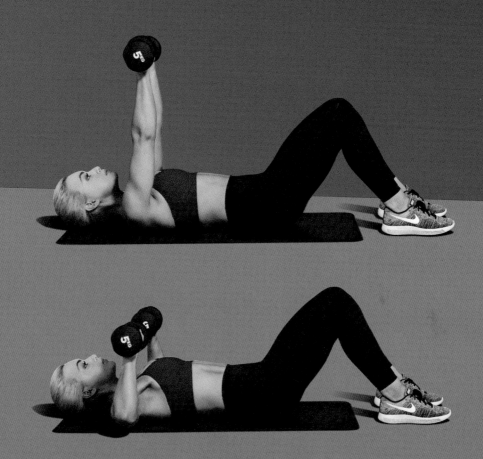

Lying flat on the floor, place your arms at right angles with the weights stable, then drive the arms up to full extension and slowly lower back down, and repeat.

UPPER-BODY HIIT (WITH DUMBBELLS)
MAN-MAKERS

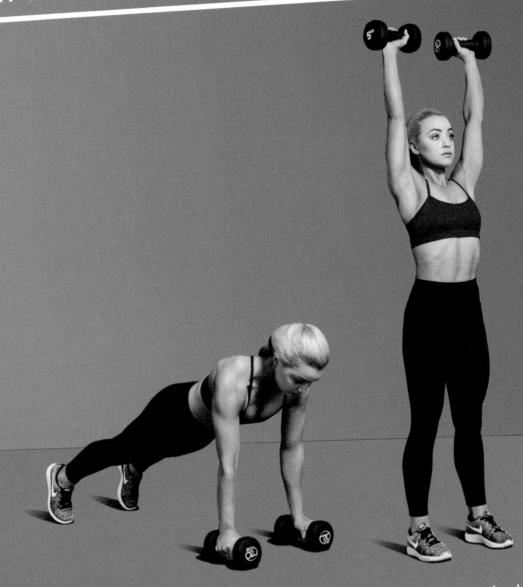

Begin in your plank position holding the dumbells. Jump your feet in towards the dumbells, then bring the body up to standing and press the weights above your head.

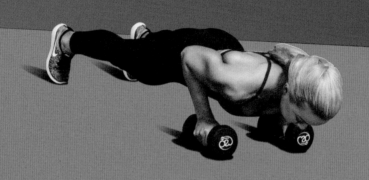

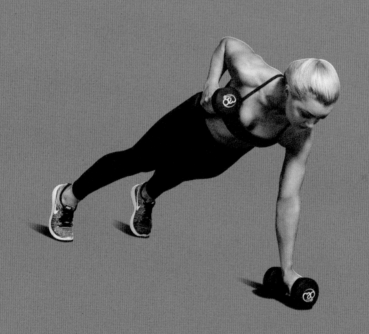

Reach down, jump the feet back out into your plank position, and then complete a full push-up, either from the knees or with your whole body before rowing either arm into the body. Once you've done this, repeat the movements again.

UPPER-BODY HIIT (WITH DUMBBELLS)
SHADOW-BOXING

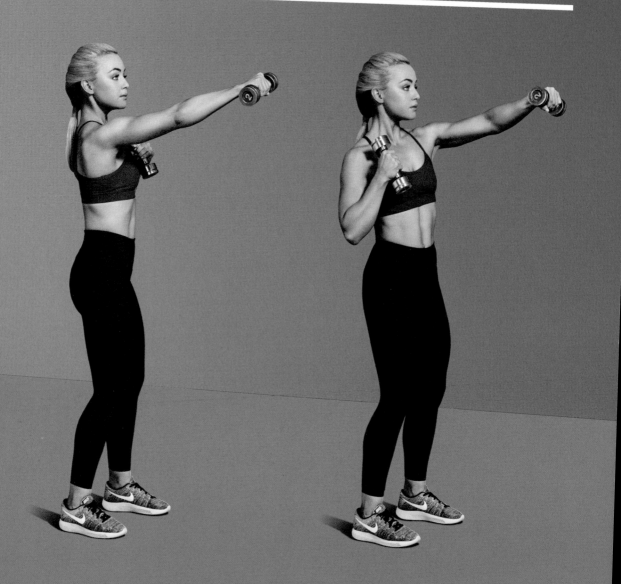

Holding light dumbells, punch one hand forwards at shoulder height, and then repeat with the other arm at a quick pace.

Love yourself first, because thats who you'll be spending the rest of your life with.

LOWER-BODY AND ABS HIIT

In this workout there is a focus on
single-leg work, designed to even out
the imbalances in strength
that all of us can suffer from
between the left and right sides
of the body, and also work on core
stability to help improve overall
strength and posture.

Complete 45 seconds of each exercise, taking 15 seconds rest
between each. Then repeat the whole circuit 3 to 4 times.

LOWER-BODY AND ABS HIIT
STEP-UPS WITH DUMBBELLS

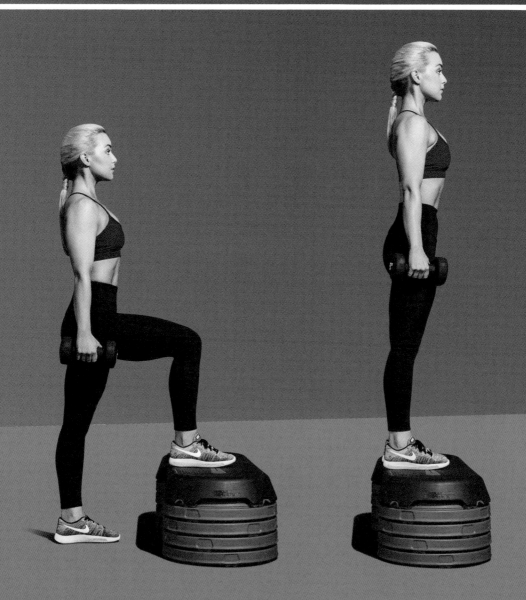

Holding the dumbbells by your side, step up with one leg onto a raised surface and step down with the opposite leg. Repeat, alternating the leg you step up with.

LOWER-BODY AND ABS HIIT
BULGARIAN SPLIT SQUATS

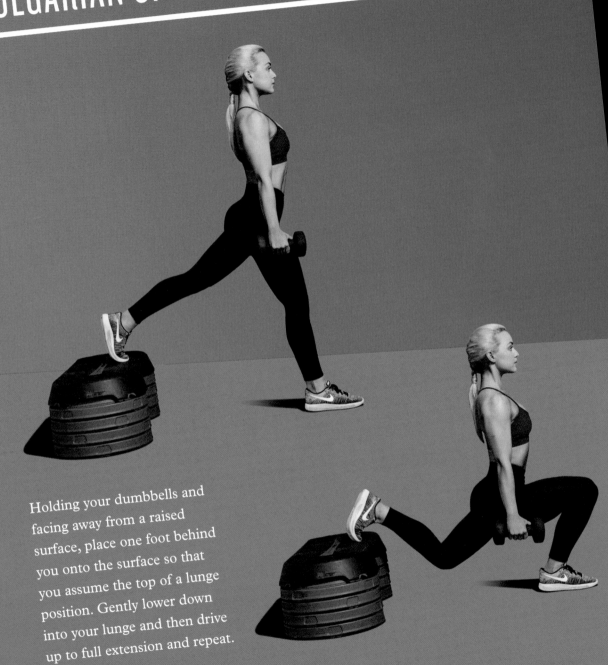

Holding your dumbbells and facing away from a raised surface, place one foot behind you onto the surface so that you assume the top of a lunge position. Gently lower down into your lunge and then drive up to full extension and repeat.

LOWER-BODY AND ABS HIIT
SHOULDER-ELEVATED GLUTE BRIDGES

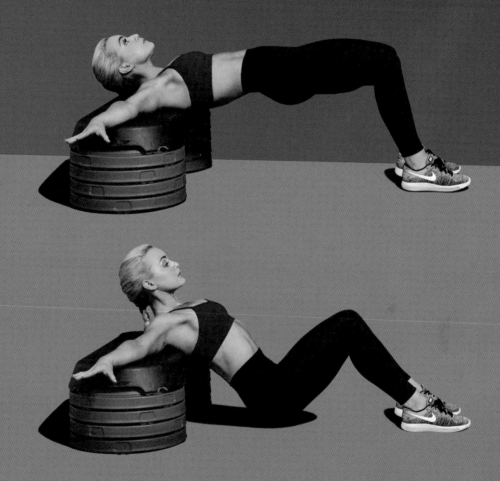

Placing the top of your back onto a bench or raised surface, walk your feet out so that your knees are bent and your torso is in a flat position. Bend at the hips, lowering them to the floor, and then drive up to your original position and repeat.

LOWER-BODY AND ABS HIIT
PLANK PENDULUMS

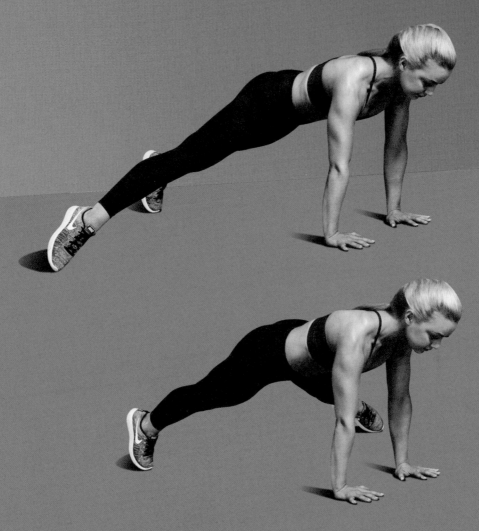

Assume your plank position. Take one leg straight out to the side of you and, as it comes back into your original plank position, take the other leg out on the opposite side, and repeat.

LOWER-BODY AND ABS HIIT
LYING LEG RAISES

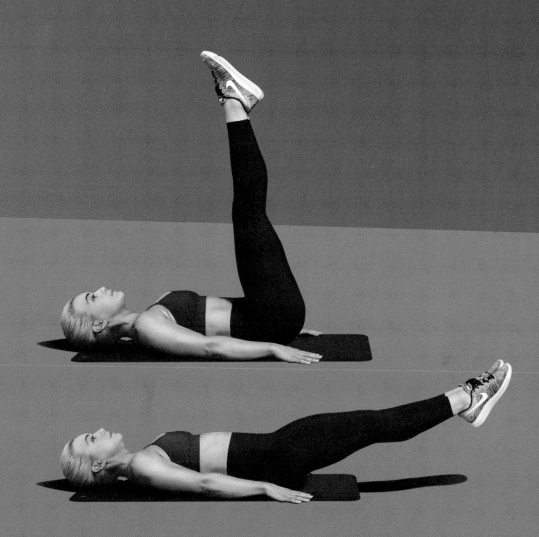

Lying flat on the floor, raise your feet towards the ceiling without lifting your lower back off the floor. Gently lower the straightened legs down to just off the floor, and then bring them back up to your original position.

UPPER-BODY AND ABS HIIT

Within this workout there is a combination of both bodyweight strength exercises and high-intensity exercises, which challenge strength and stamina. With exercises such as mountain climbers and planks it is not only the core that needs to work but the upper body also has to maintain stability, and therefore increases the demands upon the whole body.

Complete 45 seconds of each exercise, taking 15 seconds rest between each. Then repeat the whole circuit 3 to 4 times.

UPPER-BODY AND ABS HIIT
ECCENTRIC PUSH-UPS

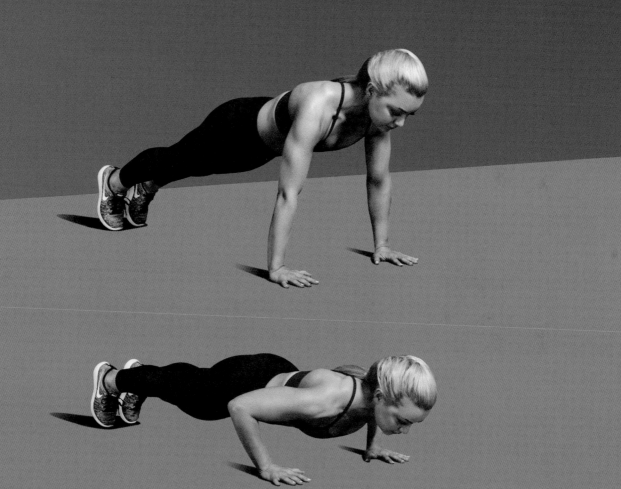

Either from the knees or from a full plank position, lower the body down slowly, taking four seconds to reach the depth of your push-up, and then drive up to full extension.

MOUNTAIN CLIMBERS

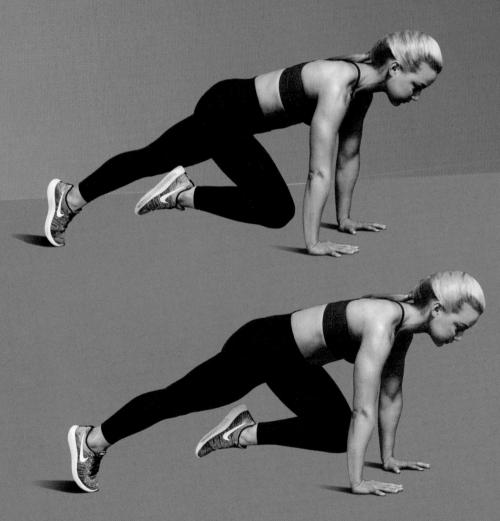

Beginning in a plank position, bring your knees into your chest alternately, maintaining a solid core and with the weight over the hands.

UPPER-BODY AND ABS HIIT
TRICEP DIPS

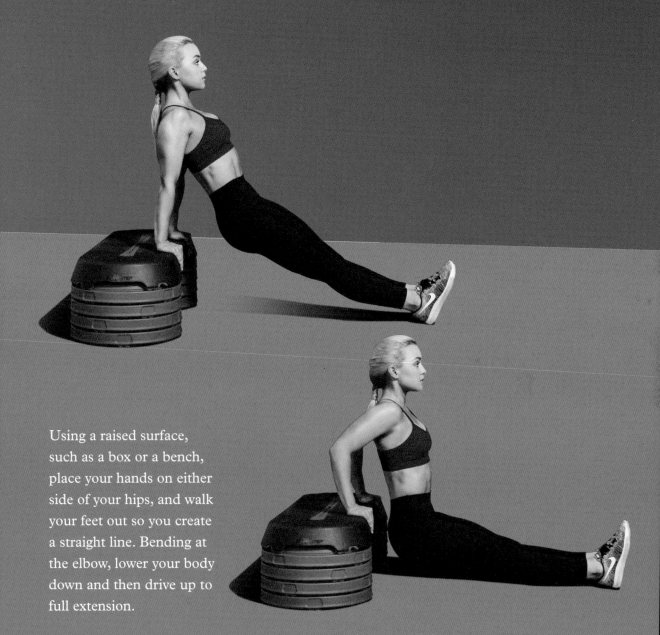

Using a raised surface, such as a box or a bench, place your hands on either side of your hips, and walk your feet out so you create a straight line. Bending at the elbow, lower your body down and then drive up to full extension.

UPPER-BODY AND ABS HIIT
BICYCLE CRUNCHES

45 SECONDS' WORK, 15 SECONDS' REST X3

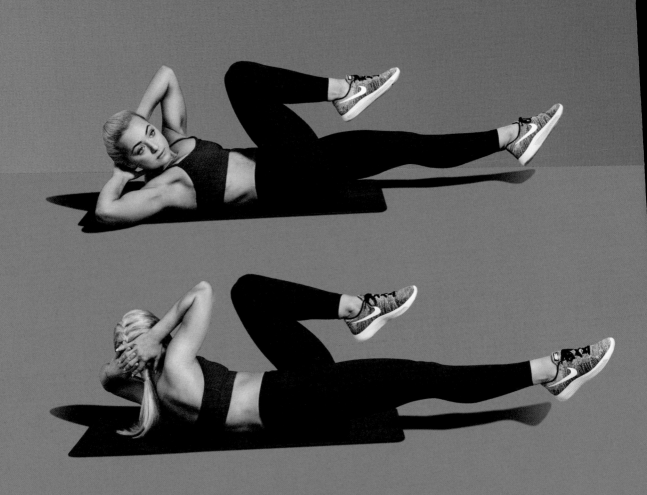

Lying on your back, place your hands either behind your head or by your temples. Bring one knee into the body and twist towards the leg, then repeat to the opposite side.

UPPER-BODY AND ABS HIIT
PLANK HOLDS

45 SECONDS' WORK, 15 SECONDS' REST X3

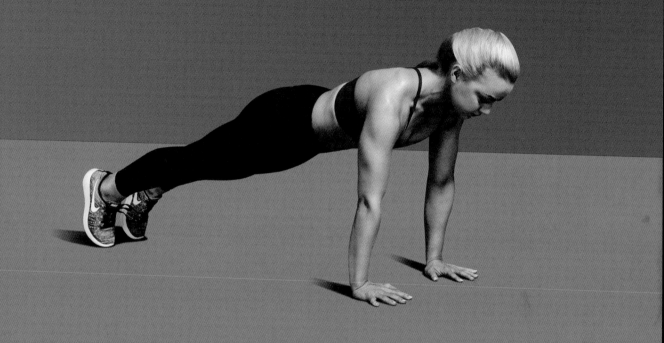

Place your hands directly under the shoulders with the arms outstretched and push up into a straight plank position, holding your core tight and with the weight over the hands.

WEIGHT-TRAINING WORKOUTS

Where exact rest times aren't indicated, I would advise taking around 60–90 seconds rest between each exercise. Don't obsess over rest times between each exercise, but being mindful of your rest periods will allow you to keep the intensity of your workout high.

For those of you who want to take your training into the gym, I am a huge advocate of weight-training and have therefore shared some of my favourite workout combinations. These will help you lose body fat and build muscle, while gaining confidence in your ability.

Before beginning weight-training it's important to set a few ground rules that will help you to train in the safest and most effective way.

FORM IS KEY: First, and something I'm incredibly passionate about, is form: this is how you perform an exercise. There is nothing more important to me than performing an exercise safely, to avoid injury and get the most out of the movement. Loading the body with weight while using incorrect form can not only be incredibly damaging, but is also most likely to be ineffective. My advice is that if you're unsure of how to do something, or if an exercise doesn't feel quite right, ask a PT or trainer at your gym, and make sure you're getting it right before you do any long-term damage.

INTENSITY: Unlike cardiovascular exercise, weight-training won't always get your heart racing or get you sweating. However, it is important to keep the intensity of your workouts high; this can be achieved by lifting a weight that is challenging, and keeping to your set rest periods. The amount you lift should be just challenging enough to complete the assigned amount of reps without compromising on form. For your rest periods, between 60 and 90 seconds is the ideal length, and while I'm not saying you need to obsessively time them, I am encouraging you to be mindful of how long you are resting between sets in order to keep the intensity of the session high.

TEMPO: When it comes to weight-training, speed is not what you want to aim for, and often rushing through sets leads to a lack of muscle recruitment and therefore a lack of intensity in the given movement. Your tempo should be slow and steady, allowing for sufficient time under tension for the working muscle group in order to achieve sufficient muscle recruitment and the correct execution of the exercise.

BREATH: Breath can be a useful tool to help power through certain exercises, and a common error I see in many of my clients is their inability to breathe through a movement, instead holding their breath. While all of these exercises require tension in certain areas of the body, holding your breath creates overall body tension which can be detrimental to a given exercise. In many instances it is best to breathe out on the resistance phase of a lift, for example when lifting a barbell in a deadlift and breathe in on the lowering phase. Play about with your breathing and find what works best for you to avoid too much tension and be able to use it to your advantage to complete certain lifts.

UPPER-BODY PUSH

When weight-training I prefer to work my muscles in opposition – that is, using a push/pull format. I do this for several reasons. First, it allows me to be more specific in my training, but you can also have more sufficient rest when you group exercises into similar movements, instead of tiring the whole upper body in a total upper-body workout. It also ensures you don't neglect pulling movements, which can often lose priority in a lot of strength-training programmes..

Within this session you work on some main compound exercises that require bilateral movement to build strength and stability through the upper body, followed by single-arm isolation work to even out any imbalances in strength between the left and right sides of the body.

If you struggle with any of these exercises, check the regression option and work to build strength in that movement before progressing to the original exercise.

UPPER-BODY PUSH
PUSH PRESS

5 x 5 REPS

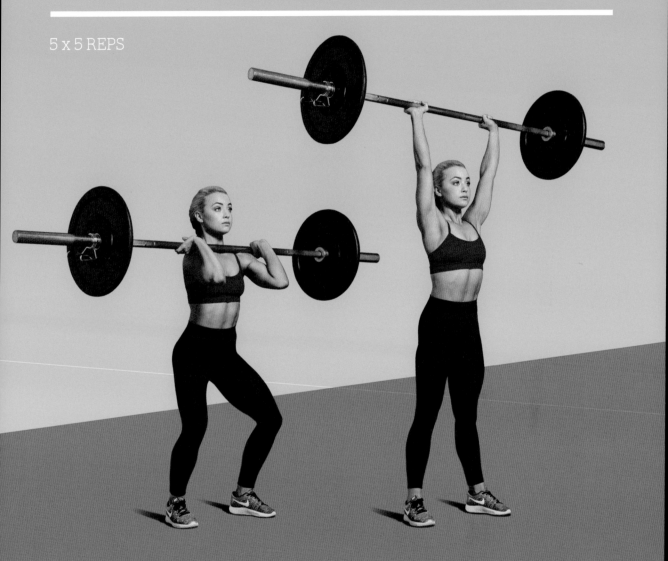

Hold the barbell with a grip that is a little less than shoulder-width apart. Place the barbell so it rests on your shoulders, with elbows high and close to your body. Bend your knees and lower your body into a half-squat position. Press the weight over your head as you press through the heels to explosively stand up.

UPPER-BODY PUSH
FLAT BENCH PRESS

5 x 5 REPS

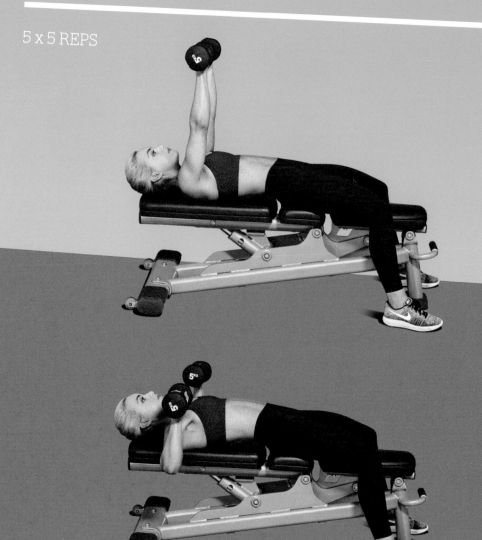

Lying flat on the bench, begin with dumbbells at right angles and then drive the arms up to full extension before slowly lowering back down in a controlled manner.

UPPER-BODY PUSH
TRICEP DIPS

3 x 10-12 REPS

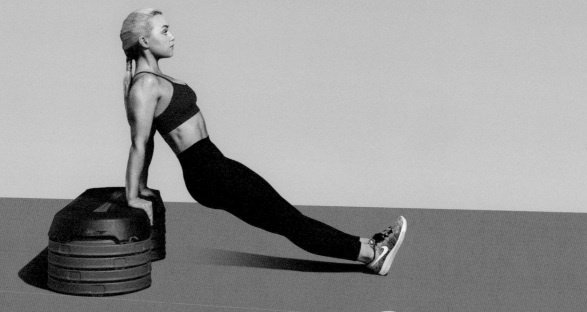

Using a raised surface, such as a box or a bench, place your hands on either side of your hips, and walk your feet out so you create a straight line. Bending at the elbow, lower your body down and then drive up to full extension.

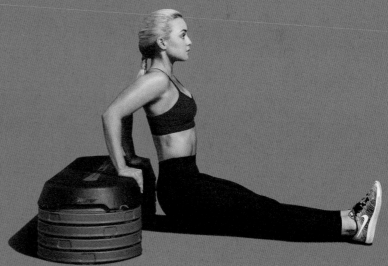

UPPER-BODY PUSH
SPLIT-STANCE SINGLE-ARM ARNOLD PRESS

3 x 10-12 REPS (EACH SIDE)

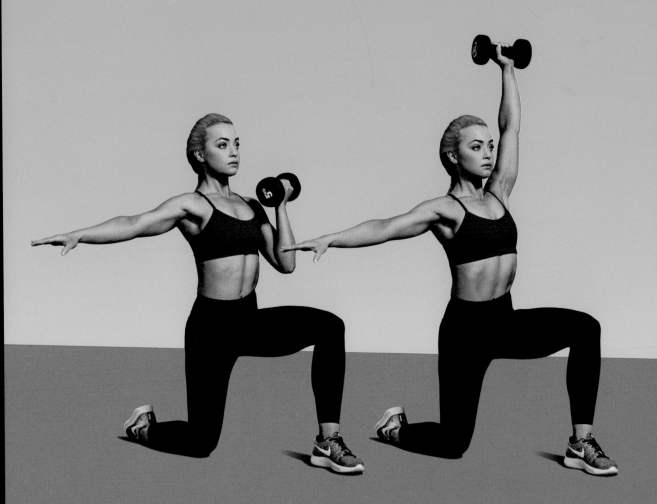

In a split-stance kneeling position, hold the weight with the corresponding arm of the knee that is raised. Hold the dumbbell tight to the body with the palm facing inwards. Rotate the weight out into a right-angle position and then drive the weight above the head, lowering it back down by repeating exactly the same movement.

UPPER-BODY PUSH
PALLOF PRESS

3 x 10-12 REPS (EACH SIDE)

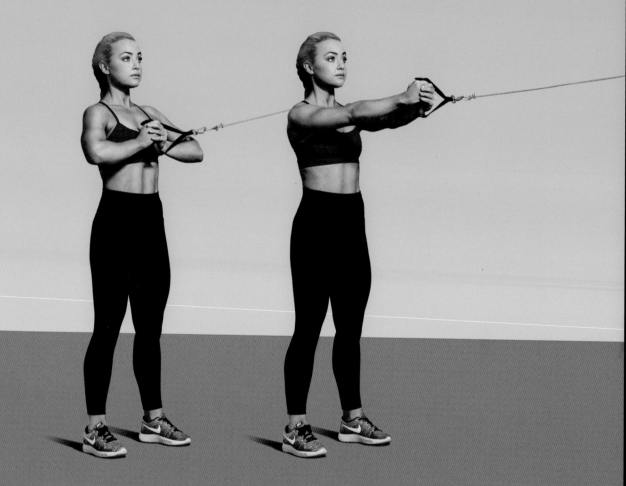

Using a cable machine or resistance band, stand side-on to the machine and pull the cable tight to the chest. In an explosive motion, push the weight straight out at chest height in front of you, and then slowly bring it back into the chest.

UPPER-BODY PULL

As a personal trainer I see so many of my clients who have desk jobs and spend hours of their day hunched over a computer. For this reason, training the posterior chain, and in this case your back muscles in a 'pull' workout, will help to improve external rotation through the shoulders to improve posture and general spinal alignment. Within this workout there is also, again, single-arm work, which not only helps to even out imbalances in strength within the body, but also encourages core stability.

ASSISTED WIDE-GRIP PULL-UPS

5 x 5 REPS

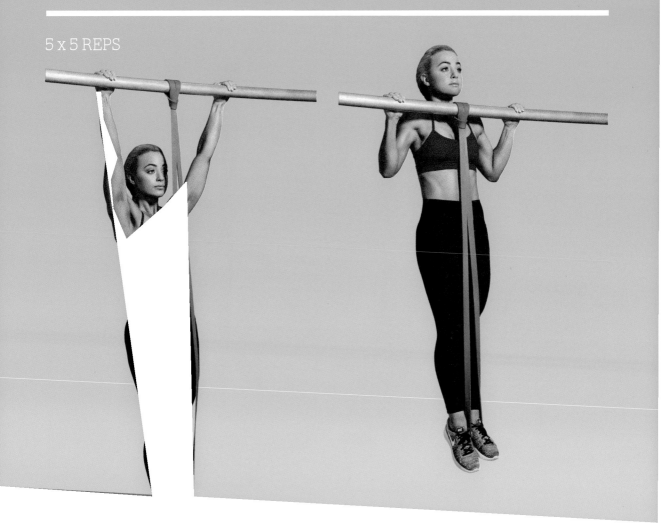

UPPER-BODY PULL
INVERTED ROW

5 x 5 REPS

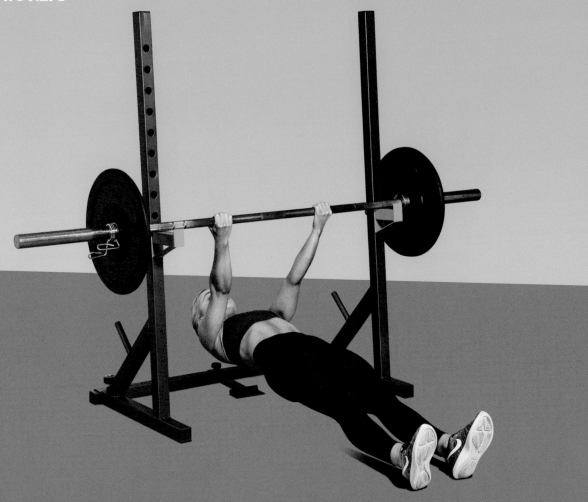

Sitting underneath the bar, take an underhand grip and walk your feet out so that you create a straight line with your body. Pull your body into the bar, aiming to touch your chest to the bar, and then slowly lower your body back down.

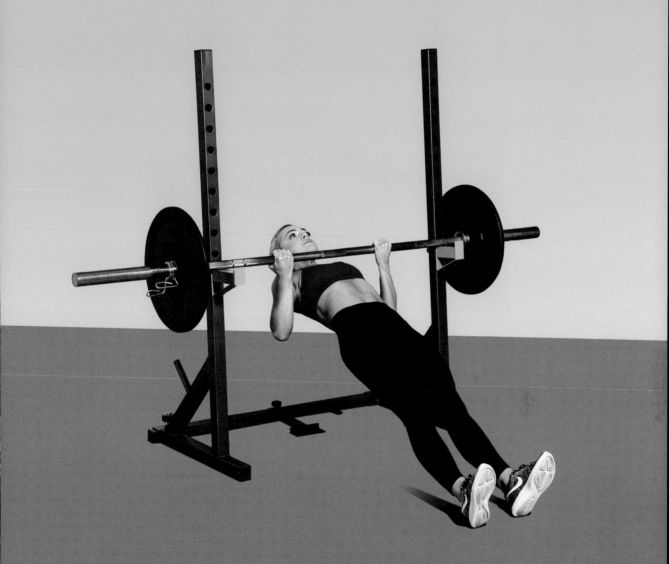

UPPER-BODY PULL
FACE-PULLS

3 x 10-12 REPS

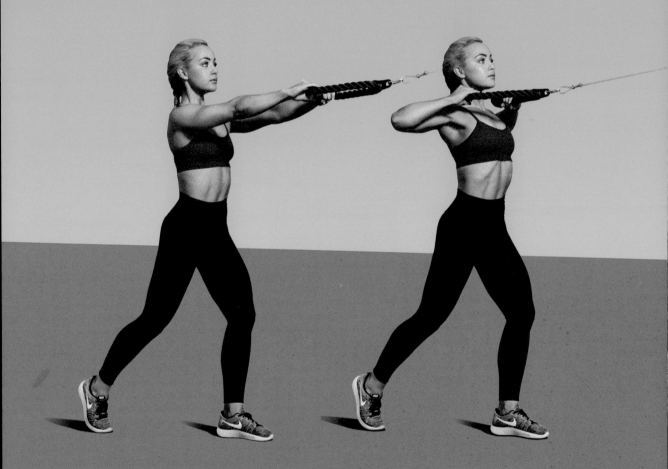

Take a split-stance position. Have the rope attachment on a cable machine set at shoulder height and take an overhand grip. Draw the weight in towards your neck, taking your elbows wide. Feel a squeeze between the shoulder blades, then slowly release the rope back to your original position.

UPPER-BODY PUSH
PARTIAL SQUAT SINGLE-ARM ROW

3 x 10-12 REPS (EACH SIDE)

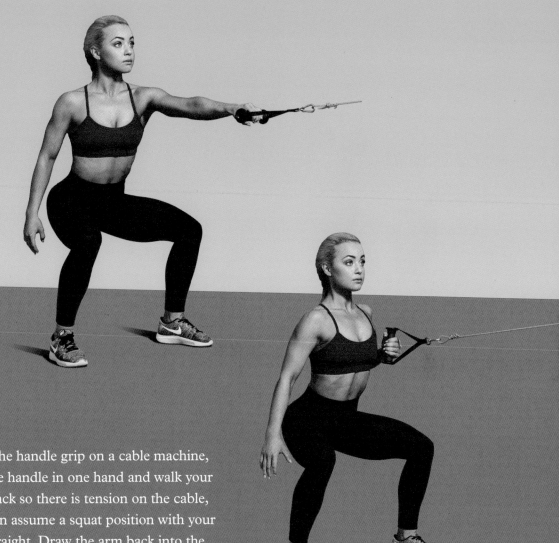

Using the handle grip on a cable machine, hold the handle in one hand and walk your body back so there is tension on the cable, and then assume a squat position with your back straight. Draw the arm back into the body, keeping the elbow tight, and then release slowly back to your original position.

KNEELING SINGLE-ARM PULL-DOWN

3 x 10-12 REPS (EACH SIDE)

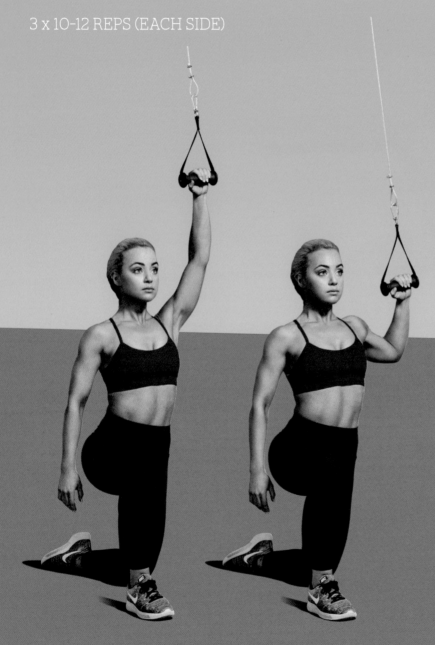

Using the handle grip on a cable machine, assume a split-stance kneeling position. With the opposite hand to the knee that is forwards, pull the cable down, keeping the elbow tight to the body, then slowly release back to your original position.

UPPER-BODY PULL
REVERSE FLIES

3 x 10-12 REPS

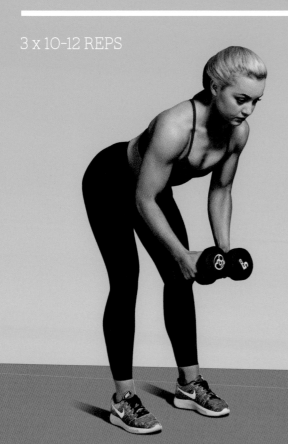

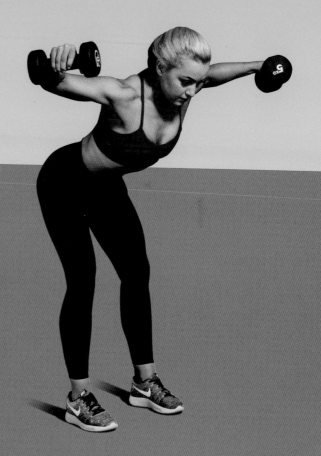

Assuming a hinged position with your back flat and your knees slightly bent, hold both weights with slightly bent arms and your palms facing each other. Then, keeping this position, draw both weights out to either side of your body, aiming to squeeze between the shoulder blades, and then lower the weights back to your original position.

LOWER BODY 1

When training legs it is always important to work on bilateral and unilateral strength, and within this workout the focus is first placed on important compound exercises such as squats and deadlifts. The focus then moves to single-leg work to challenge stability and build strength equally through both legs. Finishing the workout with an exercise such as kettlebell swings also incorporates some level of cardiovascular work to increase the overall caloric burn.

LOWER BODY 1
SQUATS

5 x 5 REPS

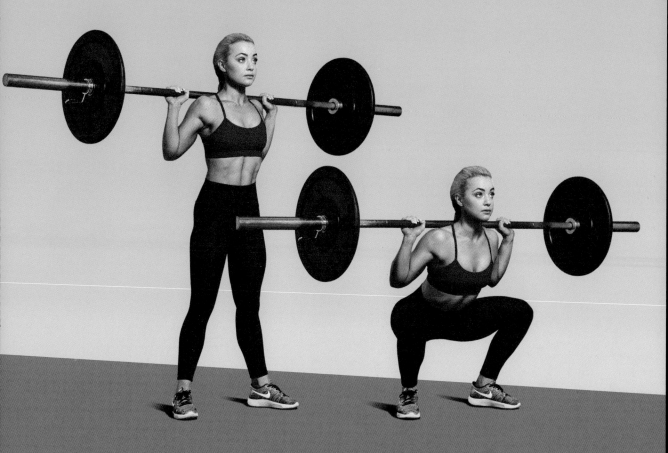

With the barbell resting on your shoulders, place your feet slightly wider than hip-width apart and then, keeping your chest upright, lower your body down into a squat position, ensuring you don't allow the knees to cave in, and then drive up to full extension.

LOWER BODY 1
SUMO DEADLIFTS

5 x 5 REPS

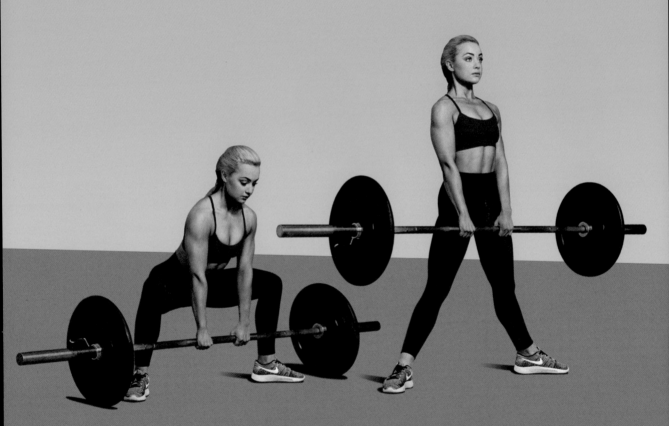

Placing your feet in a wide, turned-out stance, stand near to your barbell. Keeping the back straight, bend down to the bar, taking an overhand grip and then drive up to full extension. Make sure your hips are right under the bar before slowly lowering the bar back down, maintaining a straight spinal position.

LOWER BODY 1
BULGARIAN SPLIT SQUATS

3 x 8-10 REPS (EACH SIDE)

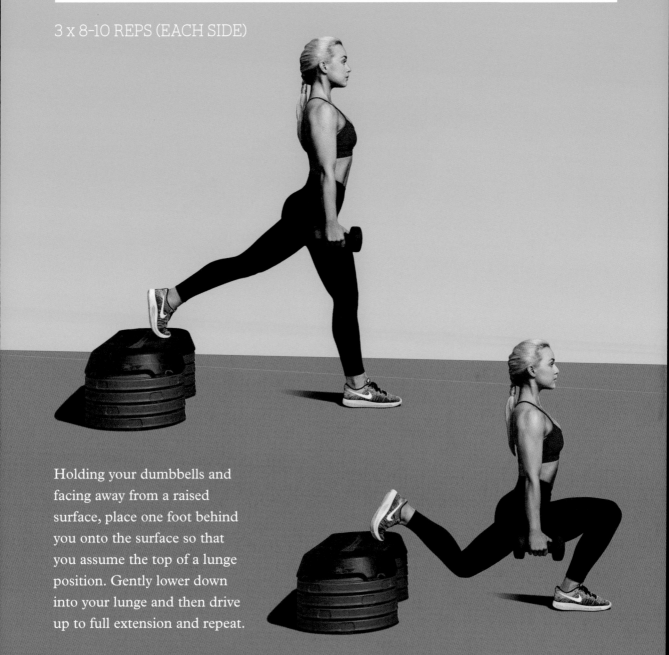

Holding your dumbbells and facing away from a raised surface, place one foot behind you onto the surface so that you assume the top of a lunge position. Gently lower down into your lunge and then drive up to full extension and repeat.

LOWER BODY 1
SWISS BALL HAMSTRING CURL

3 x 8-10 REPS

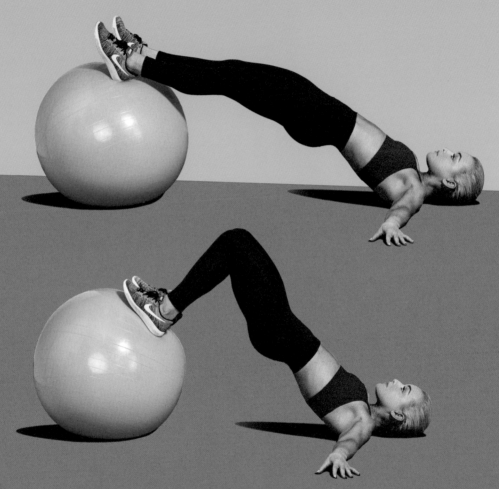

Using a Swiss ball, lie flat on the floor and place both feet onto the ball. Drive your hips up towards the ceiling so that you create a flat line with the body. Draw your feet in, bending your knees, while aiming to maintain your body positioning, then return them to their original position. Ensure your pelvis doesn't drop to the floor so that you maintain tension in the hamstrings.

LOWER BODY 1
KETTLEBELL SWINGS

3 x 15 REPS

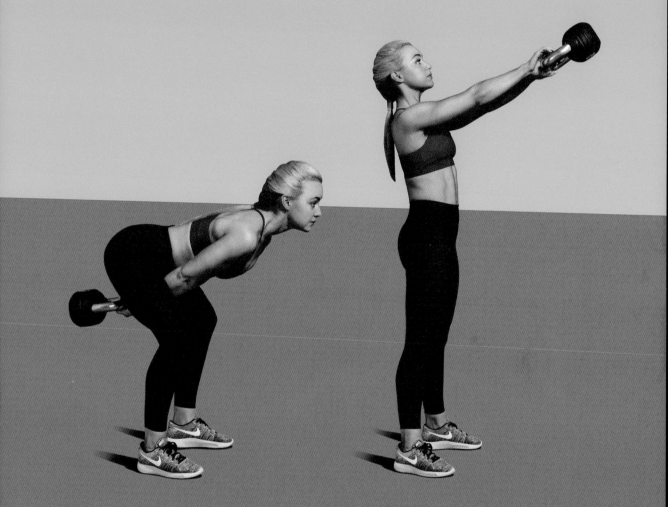

Standing upright and holding the weight in both hands, reach the kettlebell through your legs with as little bend in the knees as possible, keeping the chest upright. Drive your hips through and use the force to send the weight up in front of you, and repeat.

LOWER BODY 2

Within this workout the emphasis is placed on building hamstring and glute strength, which is something that is often neglected or underworked with the majority of my clients. There is also some progressive stability work with reverse lunges and staggered-stance RDLs to really challenge you and build strength through the whole postural chain.

LOWER BODY 2
RDLs

4 x 8 REPS

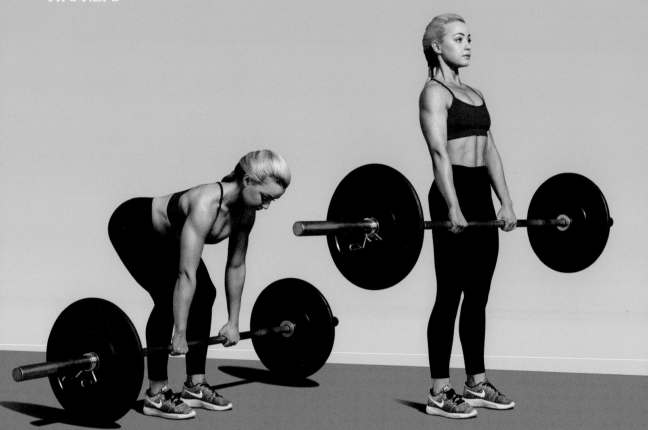

Standing close to the bar with both feet underneath your hips and toes facing forwards, hinge at the hips, keeping your back straight, and place both hands on the bar in your preferred grip. Squeezing your glutes and, keeping your back tight, drive your hips through so you assume a standing position. Once holding the bar, keep it as tight to your legs as possible so it quite literally grazes down the front of your legs, and repeat the hip-hinging motion with slightly soft knees and a straight back.

LOWER BODY 2
CABLE PULL-THROUGHS

4 x 8-10 REPS

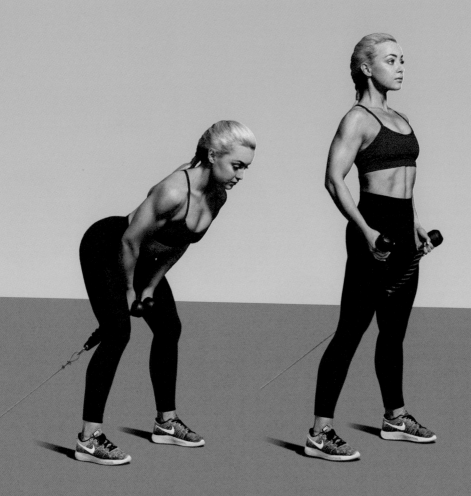

Facing away from the cable machine with the rope attachment at a low positioning, split your feet and walk out away from the machine so there is tension on the cable. Hinge at the hips and let the rope go through your legs, keeping your back straight. Then drive your hips through to standing.

LOWER BODY 2
REVERSE BARBELL LUNGES

3 x 10-12 REPS

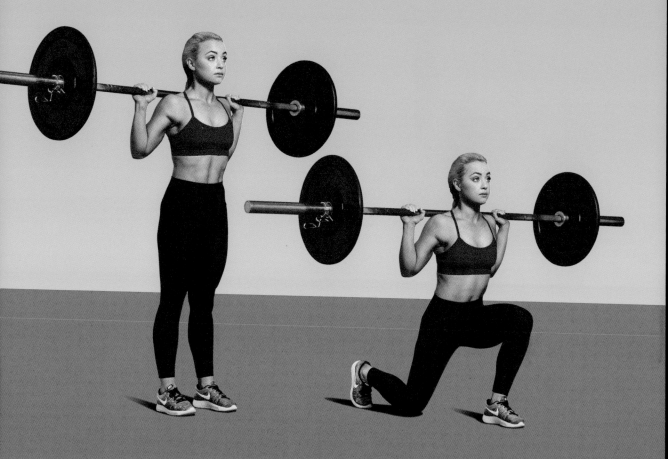

Positioning the barbell behind your head, stand in a neutral position with feet underneath your hips and step one leg back into a lunge position, ensuring the weight is evenly distributed between the legs. Drive up to your original position and repeat with the other leg.

LOWER BODY 2
SINGLE-LEG GLUTE BRIDGES

3 x 10-12 REPS (EACH SIDE)

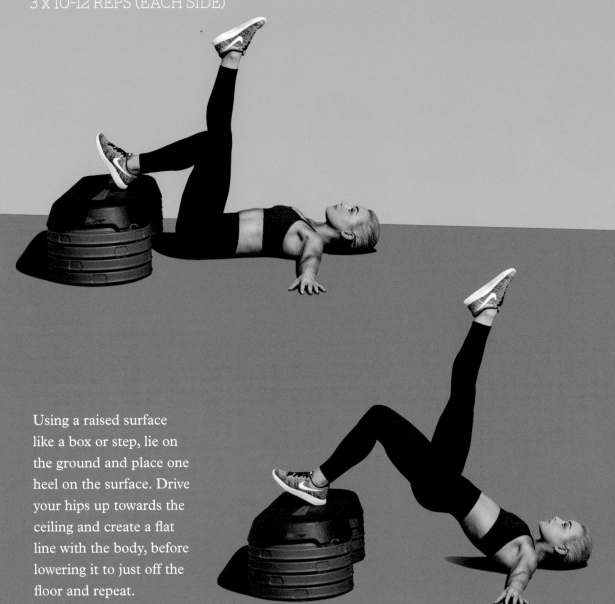

Using a raised surface like a box or step, lie on the ground and place one heel on the surface. Drive your hips up towards the ceiling and create a flat line with the body, before lowering it to just off the floor and repeat.

LOWER BODY 2
STAGGERED-STANCE RDLs

3 x 10-12 REPS (EACH SIDE)

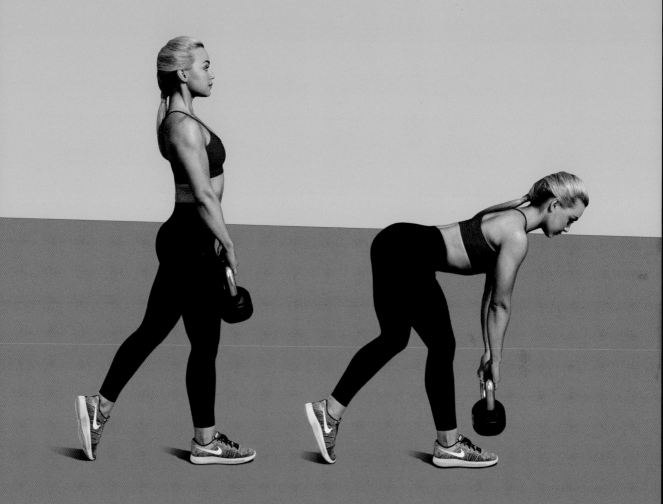

Holding your kettlebell and splitting the legs, place your weight on the front foot and balance gently with your back foot. Then, grazing the weights down the front leg, keep your back straight and hinge at the hips before driving back up to full extension.

FULL BODY

There are often times when I have little time to train, or haven't trained in a while and want a good full-body session. For this reason, I have included this challenging full-body workout which incorporates some of the major compound exercises such as squats and rows, as well as more cardiovascular-style exercises to raise the heart rate, such as kettlebell single-arm swings and kettlebell clean and press, to really work the entire body.

FULL BODY
SQUATS

3 x 10-12 REPS

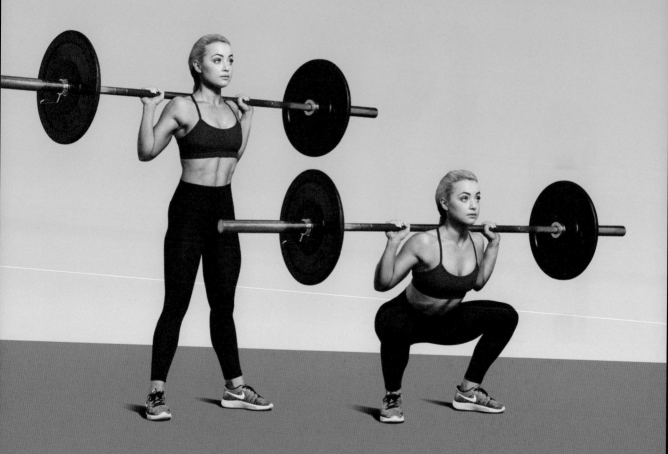

With the barbell resting on your shoulders, place your feet slightly wider than hip-width apart. Keeping your chest upright, lower your body down into a squat position, ensuring you don't allow the knees to cave in, then drive up to full extension.

FULL BODY
BENT-OVER ROW

5 x 5 REPS

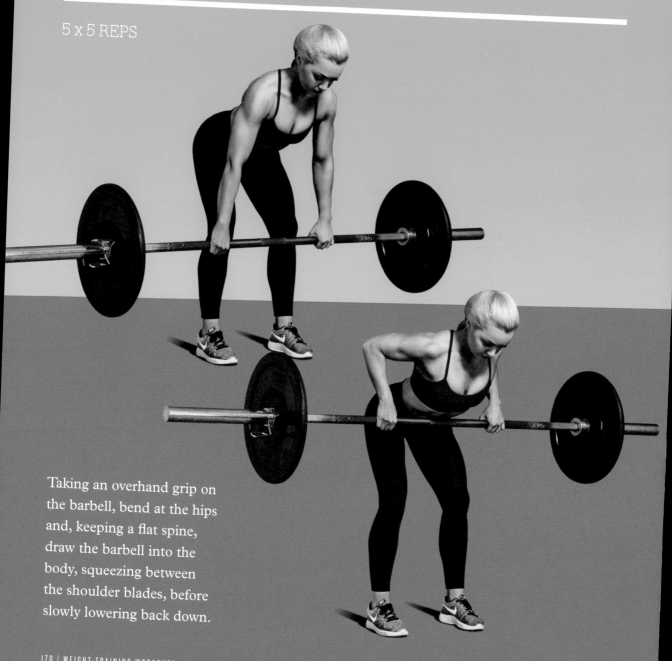

Taking an overhand grip on
the barbell, bend at the hips
and, keeping a flat spine,
draw the barbell into the
body, squeezing between
the shoulder blades, before
slowly lowering back down.

FULL BODY
FRONT-LOADED LATERAL LUNGES

3 x 10-12 REPS

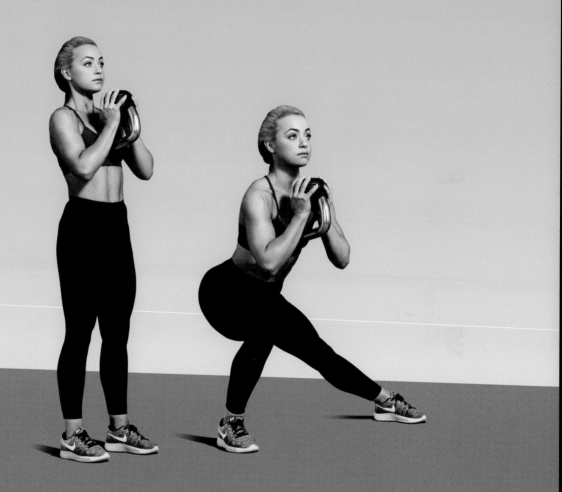

Cupping a kettlebell, stand with feet underneath your hips. Then, keeping your torso facing forwards, step one leg directly out to the side of you, keeping both feet facing forwards. Drive up to your original position before repeating on the opposite side.

FULL BODY
KETTLEBELL CLEAN AND PRESS

3 x 8-10 REPS

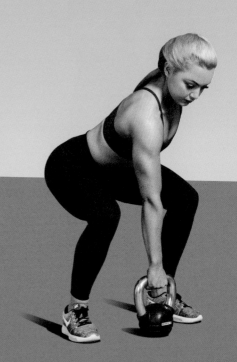

With the kettlebell in one hand, lower down-keeping your chest upright. Touch the kettlebell to the floor. Next snatch the weight up so that it flips to behind your hand and keep your elbow tight to the body. Finally, press the weight above your head, and then repeat.

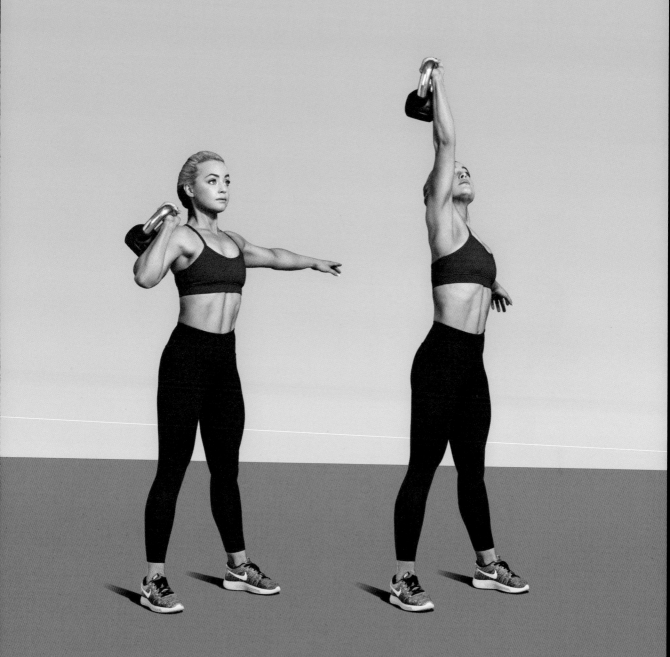

FULL BODY
KETTLEBELL SINGLE-ARM SWINGS

3 x 10 REPS

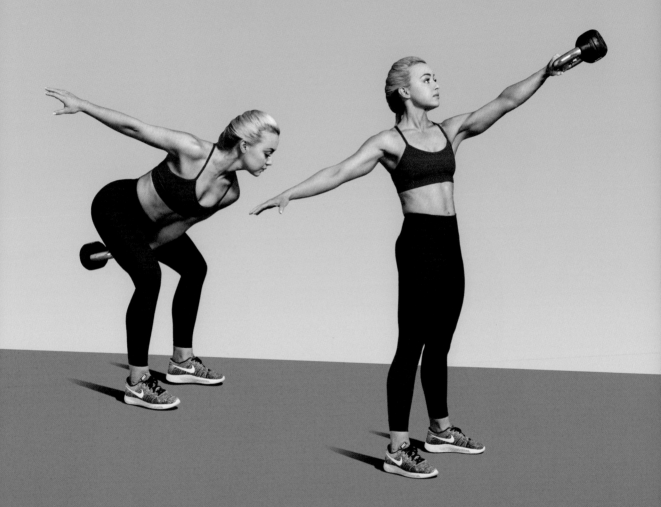

Holding the kettlebell in one hand, keep your back straight, hinge at the hips and reach the weight as far through the legs as possible before driving up and sending the weight out in front of you with a straightened arm. As the weight goes out in front of you, use the other hand to take the weight, then repeat on the opposite side.

THE BEST PROJECT YOU'LL EVER WORK ON IS YOU.

FULL BODY
ECCENTRIC PUSH-UPS

5 x 5 REPS

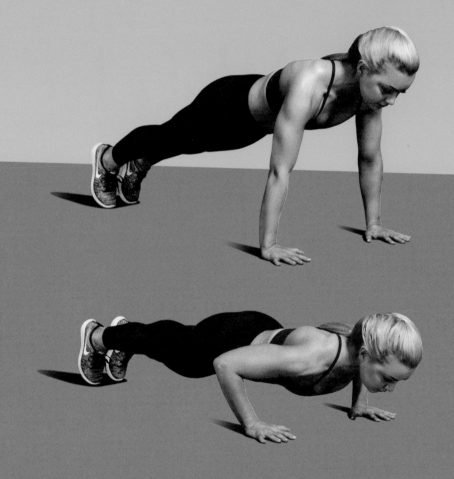

In an extended-arm plank position with either knees on the ground or in a full plank, take four seconds to lower to just above the ground, maintaining a completely flat line with the body before driving up to full extension and repeating.

FULL BODY
PLANK HOLD

TO TIME

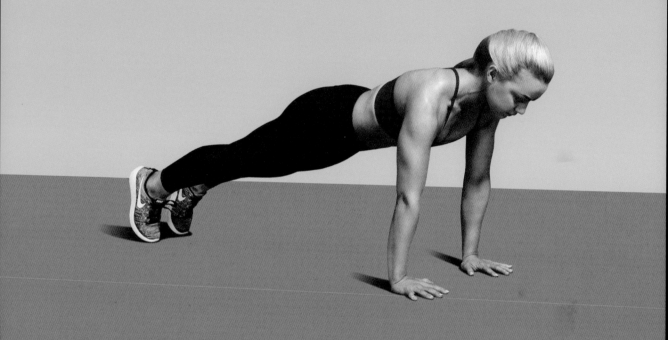

Place your hands directly under the shoulders with the arms outstretched and push up into a straight position. Hold your core tight and keep your weight over your hands.

HOME WORKOUTS

This section is designed for those of you who aren't able to access a gym. This isn't the end of the world and it's my belief that you can still have a really effective workout from home.

While on tour with the *Annie* musical there were times when I had no access to gyms or any equipment, and it was during this period that I developed ways of training that raised my heart rate but also helped build strength in both my upper and lower body. I've used a resistance band in some combinations, too, as a cheap and effective way of increasing the intensity of your training without having to get a gym membership or spend a fortune on equipment.

Where exact rest times aren't indicated, I would advise taking around 60–90 seconds rest between each exercise. Don't obsess over rest times between each exercise, but being mindful of your rest periods will allow you to keep the intensity of your workout high!

UPPER BODY I

Using bodyweight for upper-body training can be extremely effective, and just as challenging as lifting weights. The addition of the resistance band to this workout helps to increase the intensity of the workout and make it more challenging. As you gain strength, you can increase the strength of the resistance band used.

UPPER BODY 1
ECCENTRIC PUSH-UPS

5 x 5 REPS

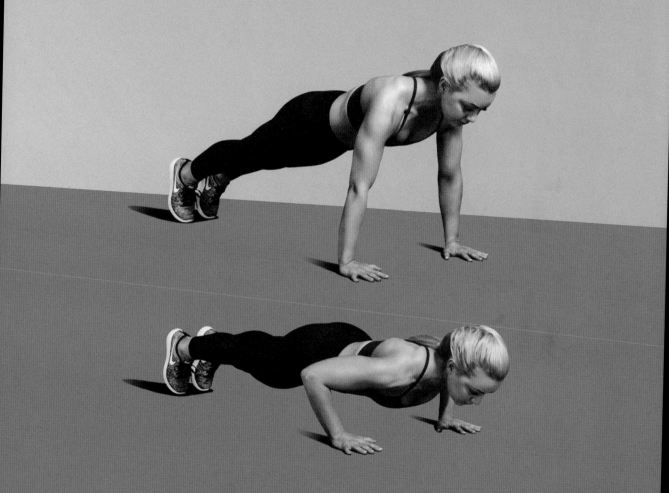

In an extended-arm plank position either with knees on the ground or in a full plank, take four seconds to lower down to just above the ground, maintaining a completely flat line with the body before driving up to full extension.

UPPER BODY 1
TRICEP DIPS

3 x 15 REPS

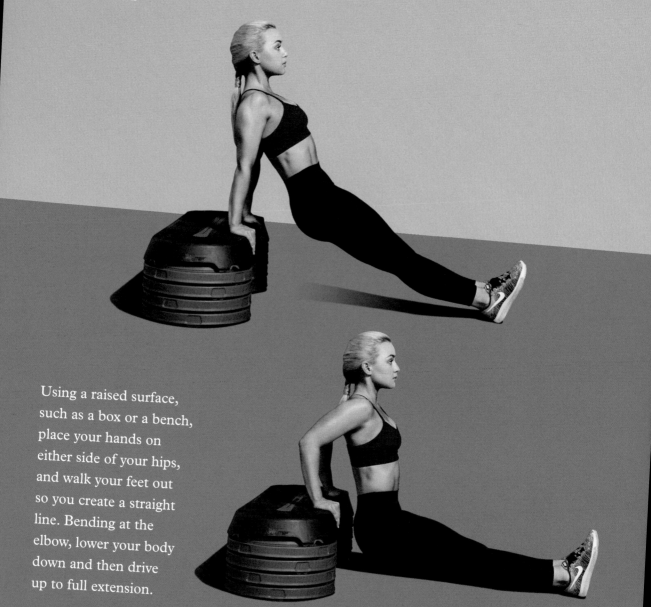

Using a raised surface, such as a box or a bench, place your hands on either side of your hips, and walk your feet out so you create a straight line. Bending at the elbow, lower your body down and then drive up to full extension.

UPPER BODY 1
RESISTANCE BAND TRICEP PULL-DOWNS

3 x 15 REPS

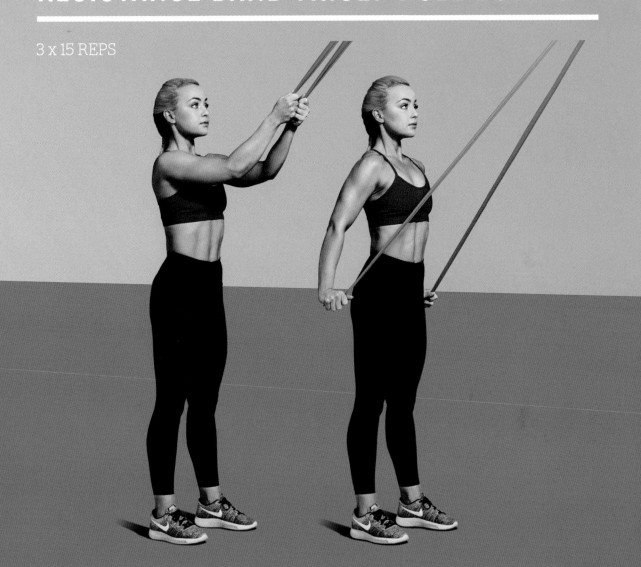

Looping the resistance band around a high object, take an end in either hand and begin with the elbows bent tight to the body and at head height. The pull down on either side, aiming to bring the band to hip level while keeping the elbows tight to the body, and then slowly release.

RESISTANCE BAND BICEP CURLS

3 x 15 REPS

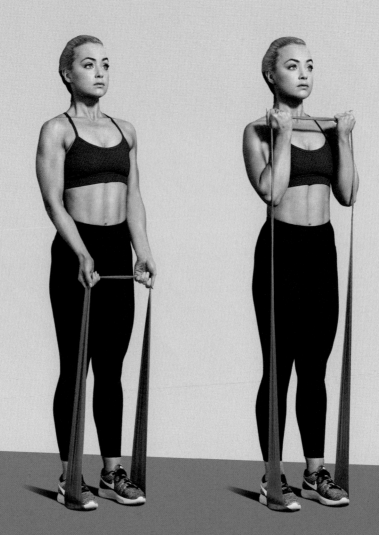

Stepping one foot onto either end of the resistance band, place both hands about hip-width apart in the centre of the loop. Contract at the bicep, bringing both hands into the body and then slowly release down.

IF YOU CAN'T STOP THINKING ABOUT IT, DON'T STOP WORKING FOR IT.

UPPER BODY 1
MOUNTAIN CLIMBERS

45 SECONDS x3

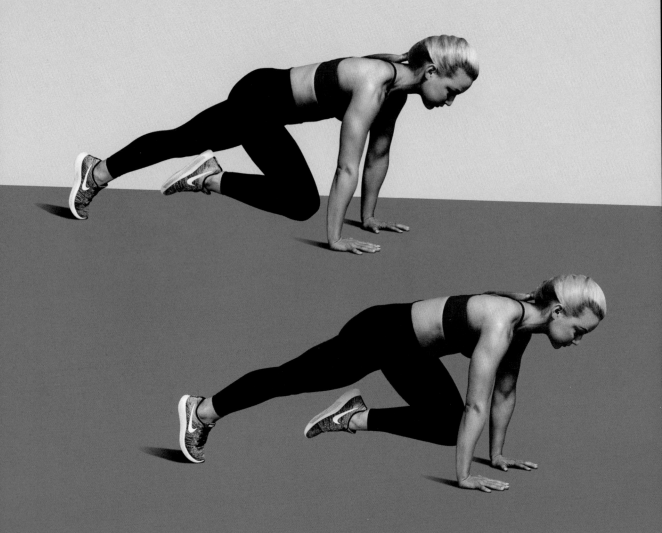

Beginning in your plank position, bring your knees in to your chest alternately, maintaining a solid core and with your weight over your hands.

UPPER BODY 1
PLANK HOLDS

TO TIME

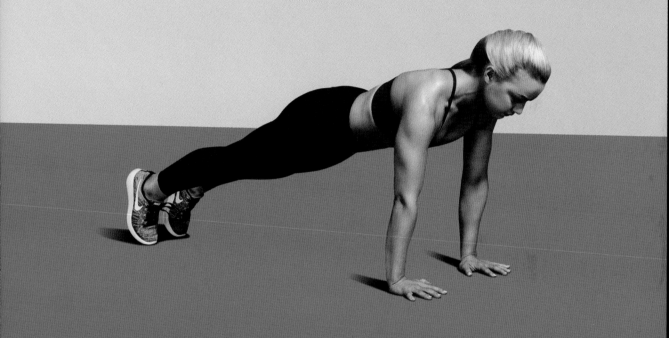

Place your hands directly under your shoulders with the arms outstretched and push up into a straight position, holding your core tight and with your weight over your hands.

UPPER BODY 2

This upper-body workout focuses on building strength through the postural chain to improve posture and overall spinal alignment. Using a resistance band helps to achieve greater muscle recruitment without requiring any large equipment, and allows you to mimic gym-based exercises such as face-pulls and rows in the comfort of your own home.

UPPER BODY 2
RESISTANCE BAND BENT-OVER ROW

3 x 15 REPS

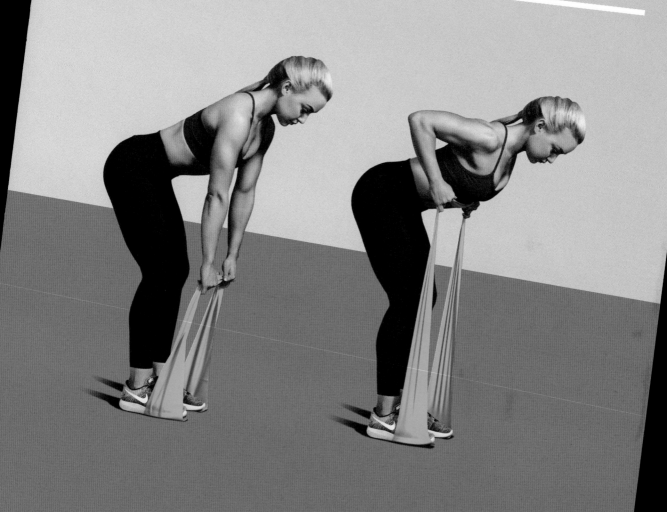

Placing one foot on either end of the resistance band, hinge at the hips, keeping your back straight, then place both hands about hip-width apart in the centre of the band. Draw both arms back and squeeze between the shoulder blades, before lowering the band back down.

UPPER BODY 2
RESISTANCE BAND TRICEP PULL-DOWNS

3 x 15 REPS

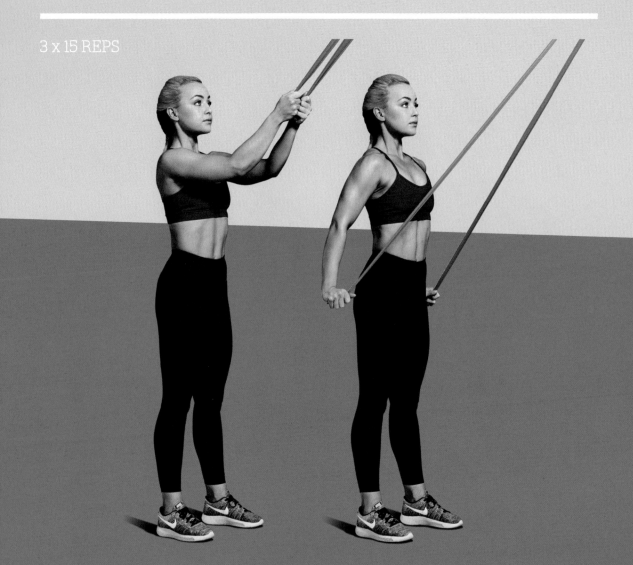

Looping the resistance band around a high object, take an end in either hand and begin with the elbows bent tight to the body and at head height. Then, pull down on either side, aiming to bring the band to hip level while keeping the elbows tight to the body, and then slowly release.

UPPER BODY 2
RESISTANCE BAND SUPINE CHEST PRESS

3 x 15 REPS

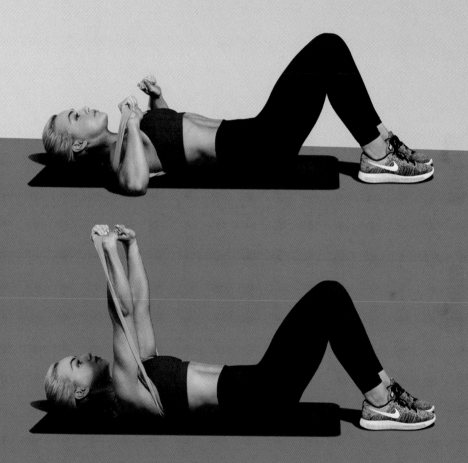

Lying on the floor, place the band underneath the top of your back, then hold either end.
Place your arms at right angles and then drive them up to full extension before slowly
lowering down.

UPPER BODY 2
RESISTANCE BAND FACE-PULLS

3 x 15 REPS

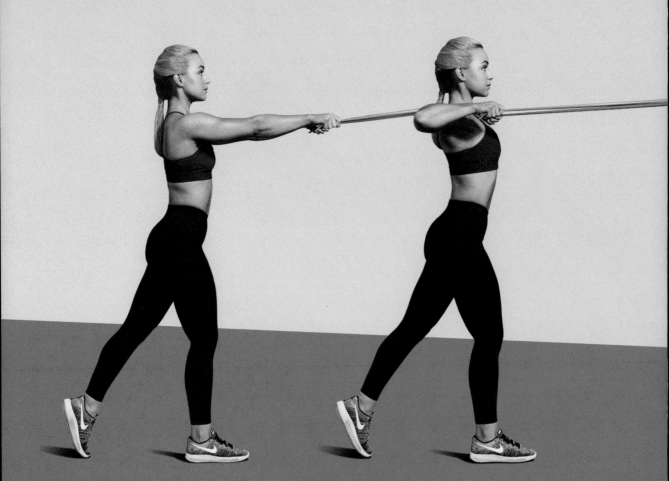

Loop the band around a high object, and take an end in either hand. Assume a split stance and, with your elbows at shoulder height, draw your hands apart, feeling a squeeze between the shoulder blades, then slowly release to your original position.

UPPER BODY 2
COMMANDOS

3 x 8-10 REPS

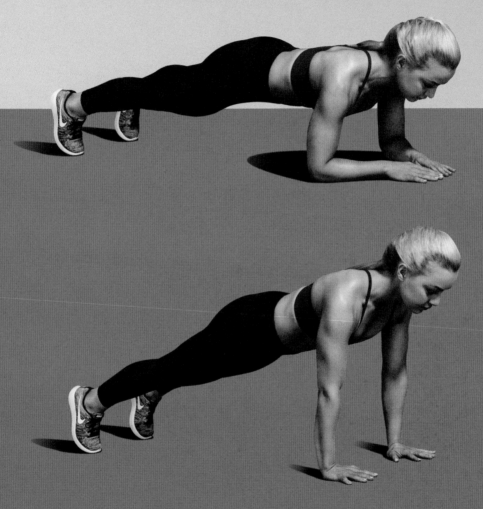

Beginning in a forearm plank, ensure your body is in a straight line before pressing up onto extended arms, and then lowering back down to a forearm plank one arm at a time.

PLANK PENDULUMS

TO TIME

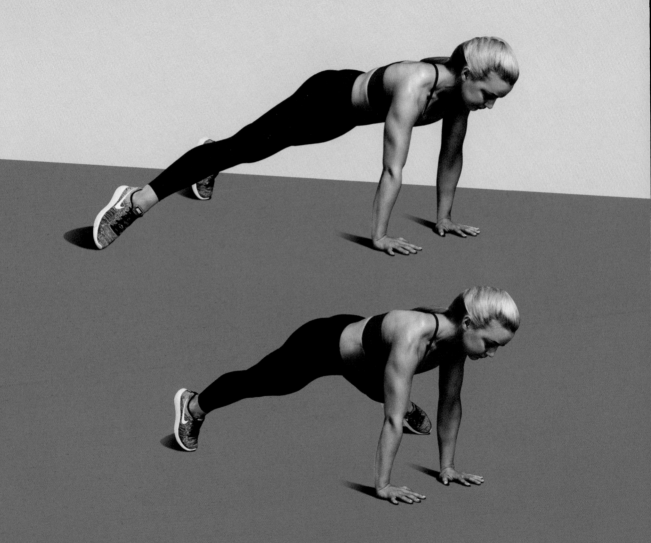

From your plank position, take one leg straight out to the side of you and, as it comes back into your original plank position, take the other leg out on the opposite side and repeat.

STOP
HATING YOURSELF
FOR EVERYTHING
YOU AREN'T AND
START
LOVING YOURSELF
FOR EVERYTHING
YOU ARE

LOWER BODY I

In this workout there is a focus on gaining strength and confidence through some of the main planes of movement such as squats and hip hinges in your glute bridge, while also working on single leg strength and stability. Having a timed exercise such as a wall-sit to finish with is an excellent way of tracking progression and gains in strength and stamina.

LOWER BODY 1
BODYWEIGHT SQUATS

3 x 15 REPS

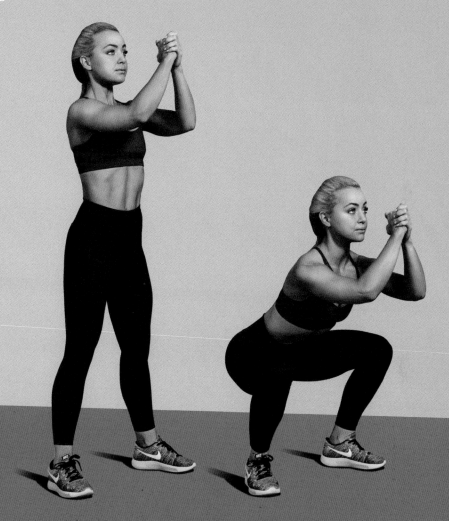

Begin with your feet wider than hip-width apart, with your toes pointing slightly out. Keeping your chest up and core tight, squat down to a comfortable position without your knees caving in, and then drive up to full extension.

LOWER BODY 1
SLIDER LUNGES TO CURTSEY SQUATS

3 x 10-12 REPS

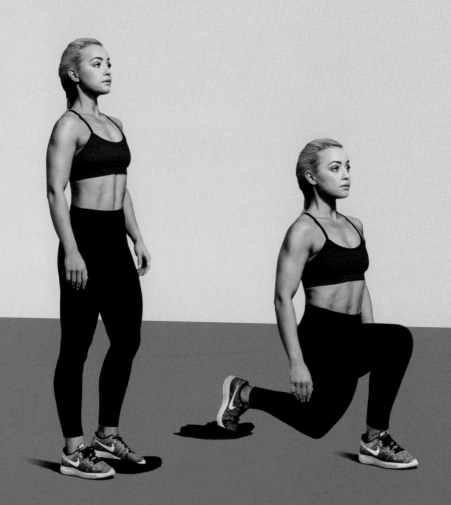

Place one foot onto a slider or folded towel. Extend the leg back into a lunge and then draw it back into a standing position. Take the same leg behind your standing leg into a curtsey position and then bring it back to standing. Repeat on the other side.

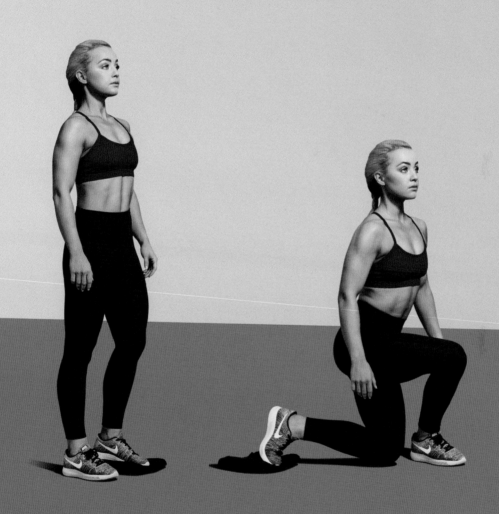

LOWER BODY 1
BACK-ELEVATED GLUTE BRIDGES

3 x 15 REPS

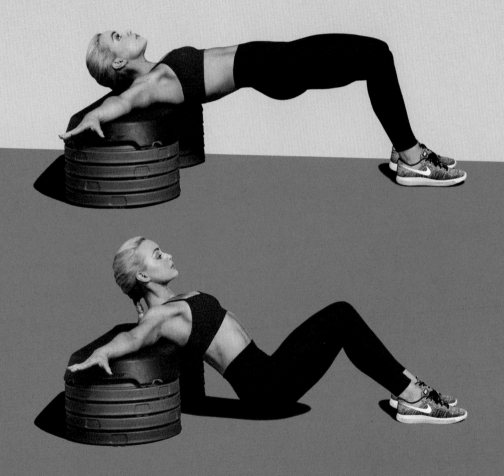

Place the top part of your back onto a chair or step with your arms outstretched. Walk your feet out to create a flat line with your torso, and then bend at the hips, before driving back up to your original position.

LOWER BODY 1
SINGLE-LEG STEP-UPS

3 x 10 REPS (EACH SIDE)

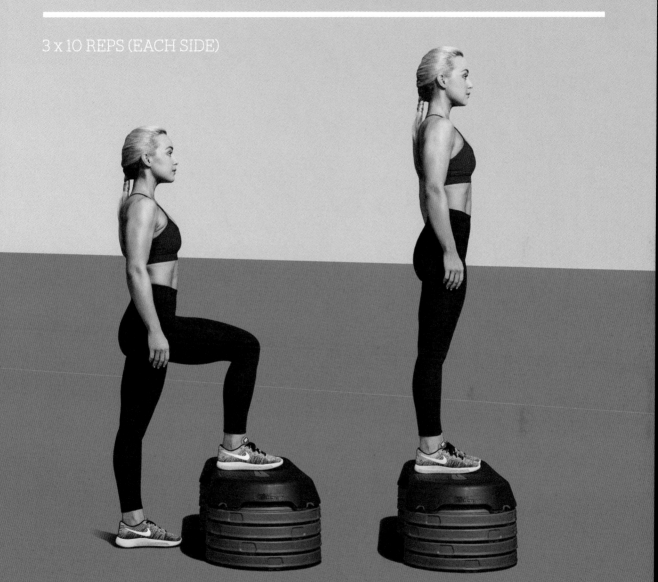

Using a raised surface such as a step or chair, step one leg up onto the chair and bring the other leg to meet it, then step back down and repeat.

LOWER BODY 1
LUNGES TO SINGLE-LEG HOPS

3 x 10 REPS (EACH SIDE)

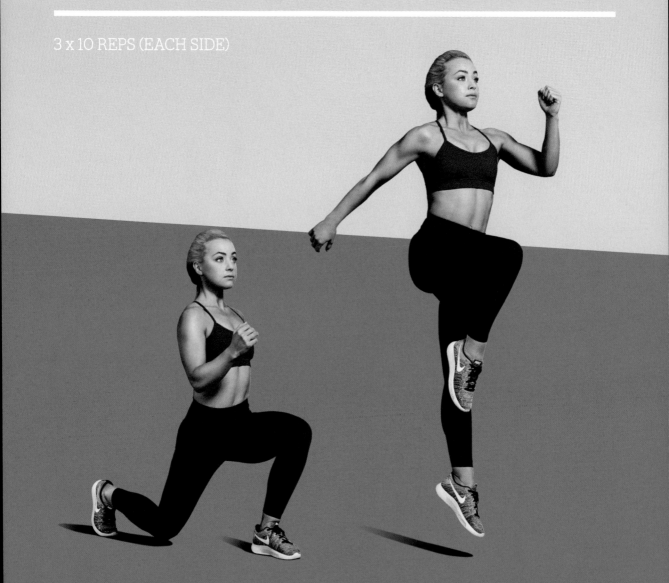

Step one leg back into a lunge, before driving up to hop on the opposite leg. Repeat.

LOWER BODY 1
WALL-SIT

TO TIME

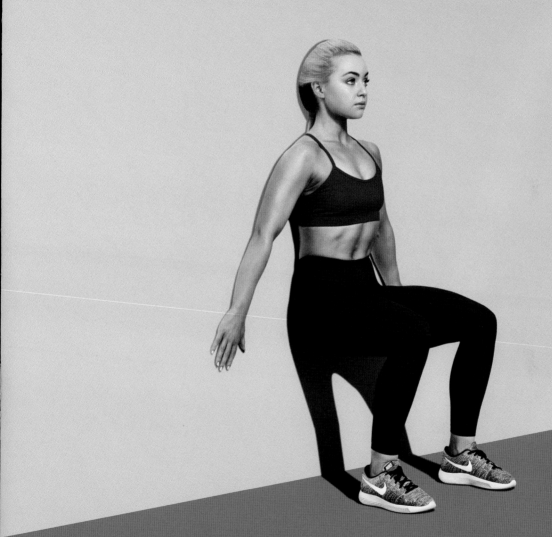

Place your back against a wall and lower your body so that you mimic sitting on a chair and hold.

LOWER BODY 2

This lower-body combination incorporates more cardiovascular-style exercises such as box jumps and toe taps, as well as more strength-based exercises such as squats and glute bridges to increase the heart rate and overall caloric burn. The addition of a full-body exercise such as mountain climbers also ensures you've got a total body burner to finish the circuit to really challenge you!

LOWER BODY 2
PRISONER SQUATS

3 x 15 REPS

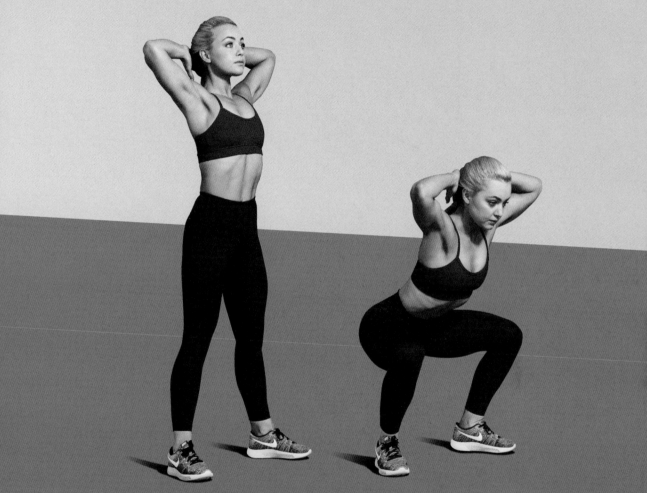

Place both hands behind the head with fingers interlaced. Keeping your chest up, take your feet slightly turned out and a little wider than hip-width apart. Squat down and drive up to full extension.

LOWER BODY 2
BACK-ELEVATED GLUTE BRIDGES

3 x 15 REPS

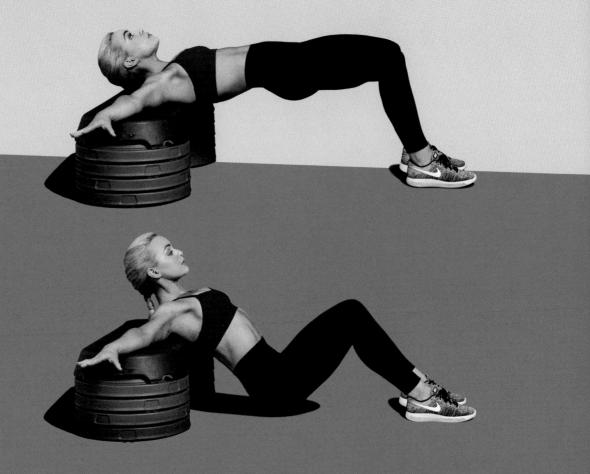

Place the top part of your back onto a chair or step with your arms outstretched. Walk your feet out to create a flat line with your torso, and then bend at the hips, before driving back up to your original position.

LOWER BODY 2
SINGLE-LEG GLUTE BRIDGES

3 x 10 REPS (EACH SIDE)

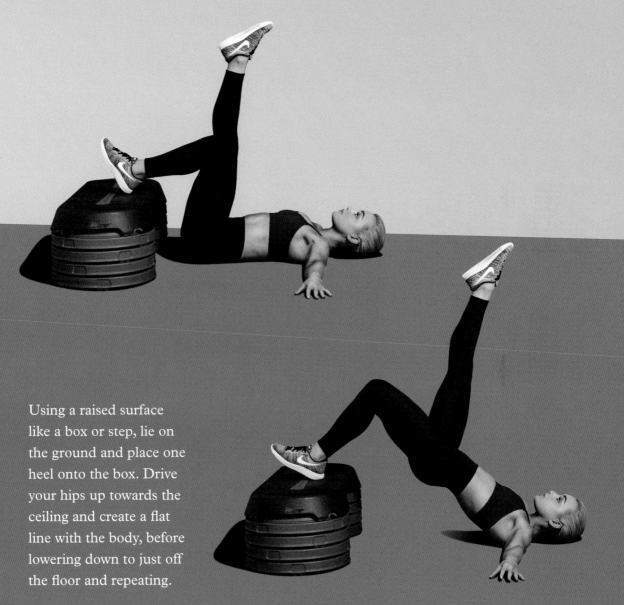

Using a raised surface like a box or step, lie on the ground and place one heel onto the box. Drive your hips up towards the ceiling and create a flat line with the body, before lowering down to just off the floor and repeating.

LOWER BODY 2
TOE TAPS

45 SECONDS X 3

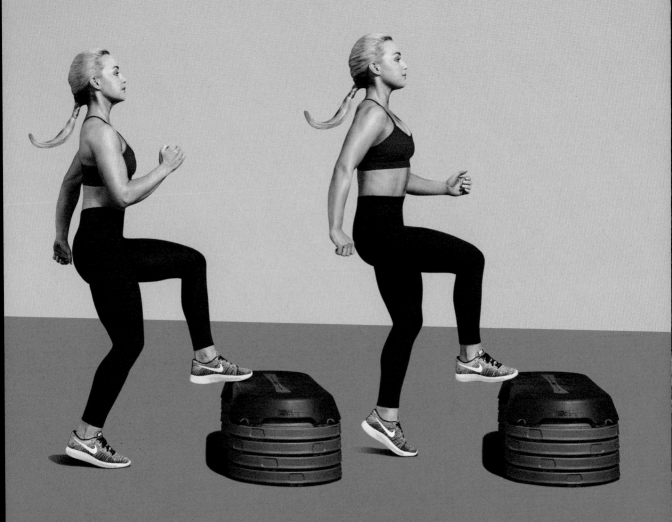

Using a raised surface such as a step, in a jumping motion tap either foot onto the step, using your arms to power you.

LOWER BODY 2
BOX JUMPS

45 SECONDS X 3

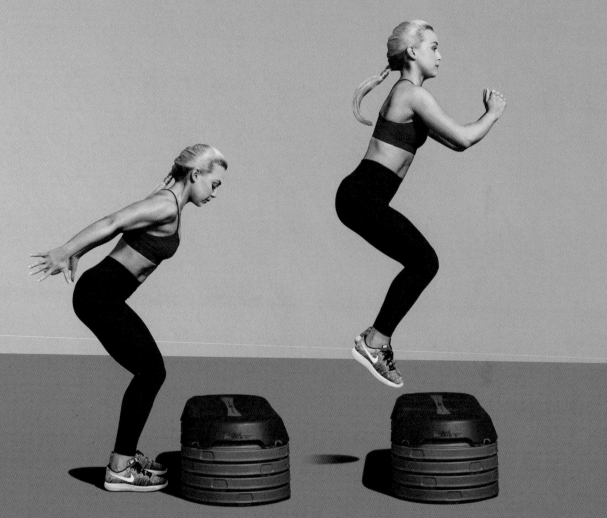

Using a sturdy box or step, jump from both feet onto the box and then step down, and repeat.

LOWER BODY 2
MOUNTAIN CLIMBERS

45 SECONDS X 3

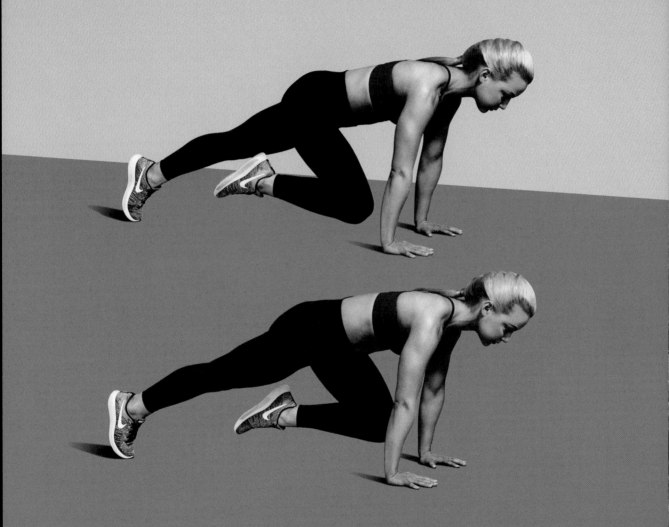

Beginning in a plank position, bring your knees into your chest alternately, maintaining a solid core with the weight over the hands.

I'M WORKING ON MYSELF, FOR MYSELF, BY MYSELF.

FULL BODY

For those days when you require a real full-body workout, this combination will not only raise your heart rate and get you sweating, but also challenge plyometric (jump-training) strength with exercises such as ski jumps and plyometric lunges, as well as strength-based exercises such as plank holds.

FULL BODY
SKI JUMPS

3 x 20 REPS

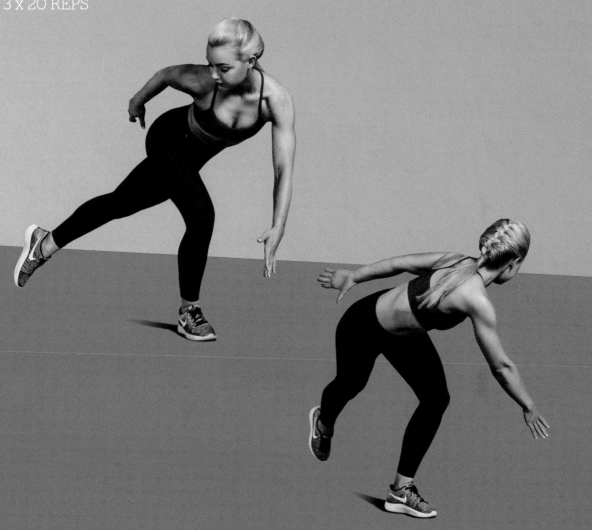

From standing, jump laterally onto one leg, taking the other off the floor and behind the standing leg, twisting the body towards the leg, then repeat on the opposite side.

FULL BODY
COMMANDOS

45 SECONDS X 3

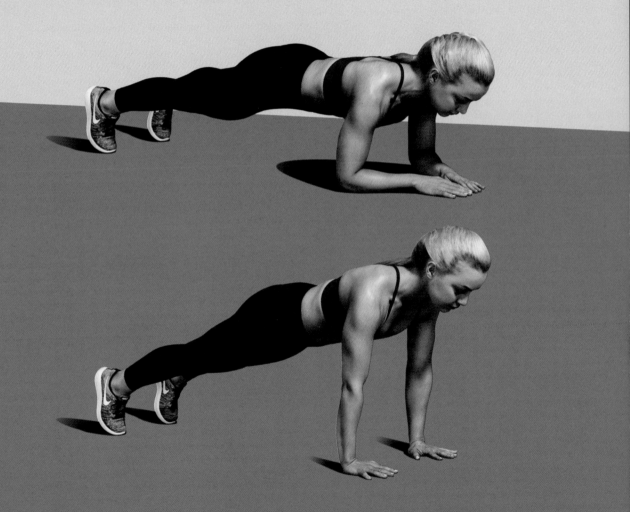

Beginning in a forearm plank, ensure your body is in a straight line before pressing up onto extended arms, and then lower back down to a forearm plank one arm at a time, and repeat.

FULL BODY
PLYOMETRIC LUNGES

3 X 20 REPS

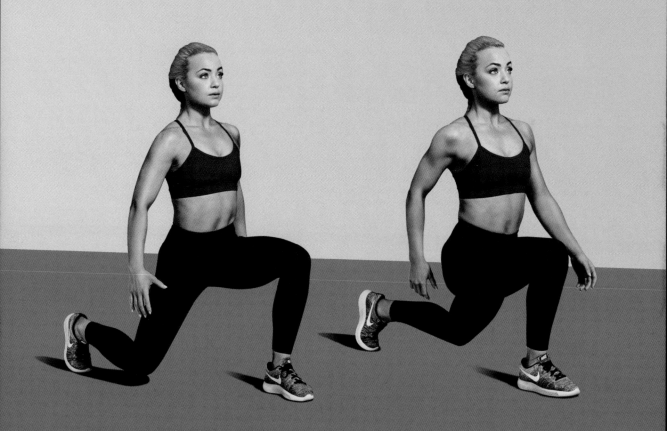

Assume the bottom of a lunge position and then, using your arms, jump up into the air and switch legs; repeat.

FULL BODY
BURPEES

3 x 10 REPS

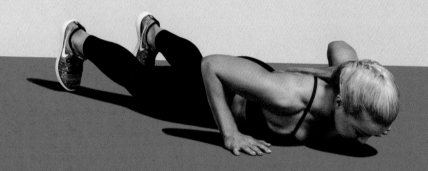

Begin with your chest touching the floor and your arms bent with your hands at either side of your body.

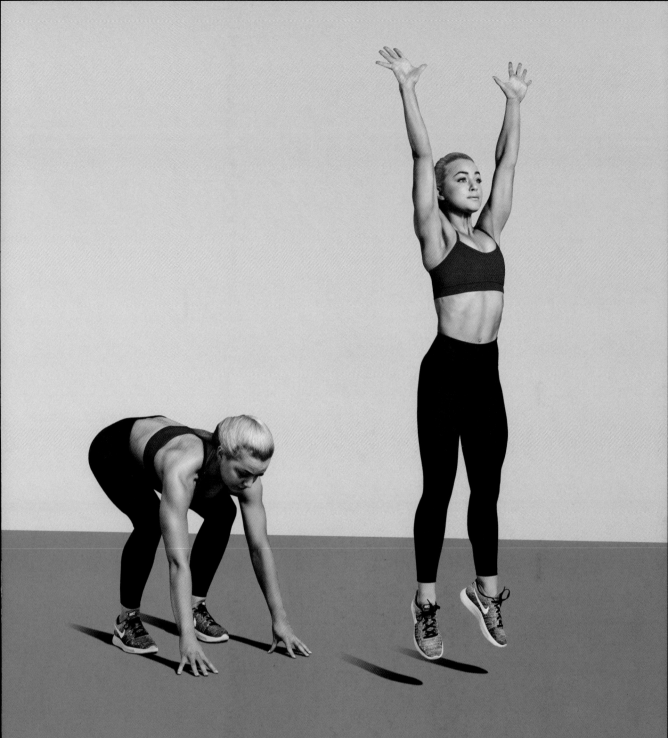

Jump your feet in, and jump up into the air before placing your hands back on the floor and assuming your original position; repeat.

FULL BODY
ECCENTRIC PUSH-UPS

5 x 5 REPS

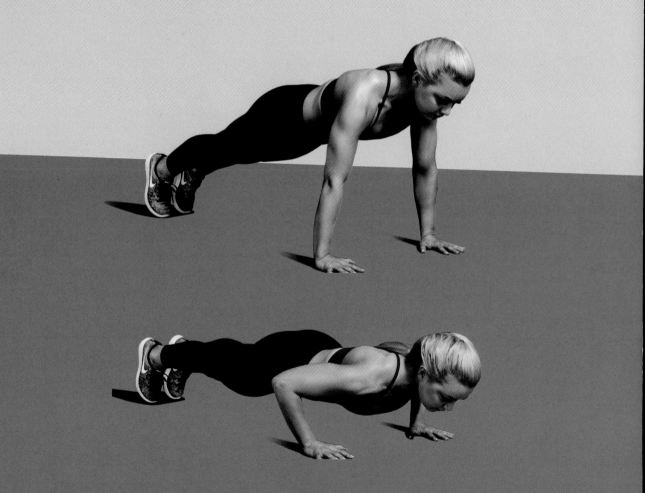

Either from the knees or from a plank position, lower your body down slowly, taking four seconds to reach the depth of your push-up, then drive up to full extension.

FULL BODY
PLANK HOLDS

TO TIME

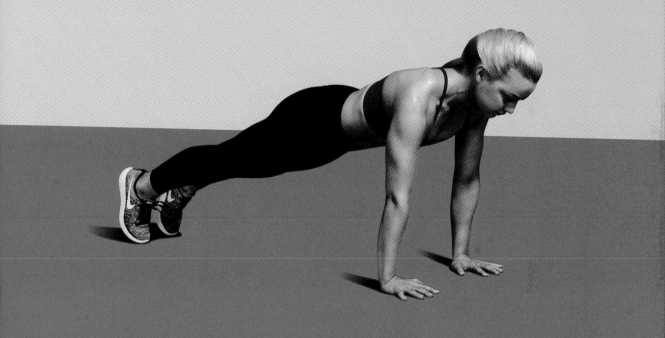

Place your hands directly under your shoulders with your arms outstretched and push up into a straight position, holding your core tight and with the weight over the hands.

360° RECOVERY

In this section of the book I want to impress upon you the importance of not just viewing your training in isolation, but looking instead at the bigger picture so that you can ensure your recovery is as good as possible to support your fitness regime. Neglecting aspects of your whole-body recovery is detrimental to your overall health and will deter you from achieving your goals.

I believe we should see our bodies as a 360° picture of health, which involves being aware of all aspects of the small building blocks that come together to create the happiest and healthiest version of yourself.

SLEEP:

One of the most overlooked aspects of exercise recovery is sleep, both its quantity and quality. A lack of sleep, or a lack of good-quality sleep, can lead to a decrease in cognitive function and an increase in stress levels, and can affect things such as your appetite for food. All of these will dramatically impact on your motivation to maintain your exercise programme.

Many studies have shown the benefits of exercise on the quality and length of your sleep, and a decrease in either the amount of sleep you get or its quality can mean that your muscles aren't given a chance to fully repair. There is no hard-and-fast rule about how many hours of sleep a night you need to be getting, but I find that it should generally be around eight hours. If you are constantly waking up feeling tired, the chances are you're not getting enough!

There are many ways in which you can aim to improve your sleep quality, and below I've listed a few of my top tips. It's worth mentioning that if you are really suffering from lack of sleep I'd recommend speaking to a health professional such as your GP.

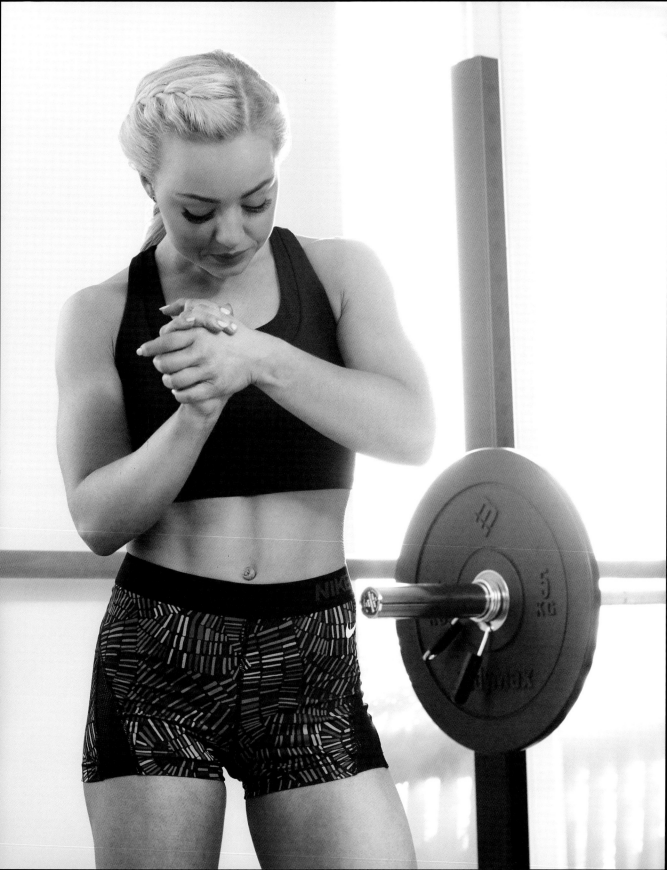

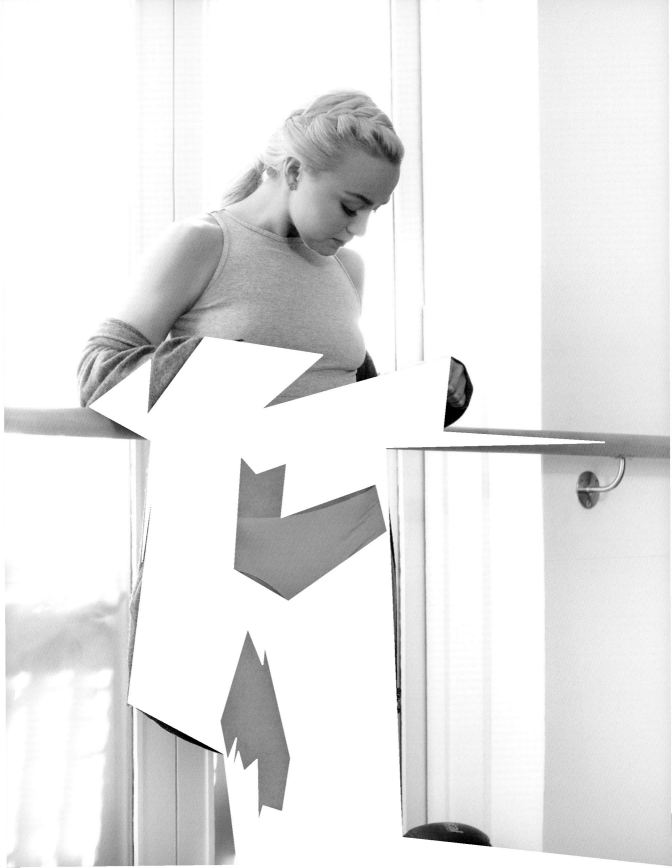

MY TOP TIPS FOR A SOUND NIGHT'S SLEEP

1. Don't let stress overwhelm you before bed. If you've got lots on your mind, try writing it down before you sleep as this will help to clear your mind.

2. Have a night-time routine. Allow your body the chance to mentally prepare for sleep by having a consistent routine you follow every night before bed. Whether it's a bath, shower or reading a book, it should be calming and give you some head space to wind down.

3. Cut the caffeine. If you're finding it difficult to drop off, try reducing your caffeine intake, particularly in the afternoon and evening, and see if this helps.

4. Switch it off. Lying in bed and looking at your phone or your laptop, or watching TV, stimulates your brain and does the opposite to preparing your body for sleep. Aim to have all electrical equipment off and on silent around 20 to 30 minutes before you go to sleep to give your body a chance to settle.

5. Read a book! Something I find helps prepare me for bed is reading. Find a good book, in any genre that interests you, and aim to read at least ten pages before bed.

STRESS

The 21st century can be a stressful time in which to live, and it's a challenge not to feel the pressure in our day-to-day lives. Stress cannot be avoided in many situations, but consistently elevated stress levels can cause an increase in the release of the hormone cortisol. This provides the body with glucose, and can therefore lead to increased blood sugar levels. In addition to this, multiple studies have shown stress to be linked to things such as increased fatigue, poor quality of sleep, high blood pressure or hypertension, and general irritability. All of these are not helpful to improving our health and happiness, and therefore it's extremely important to learn to control your stress levels. Here are some of my favourite stress-busting tips to help you manage stress:

1. Make a list. I often get the overwhelming feeling of having too much to do, and simply writing down what I need to do in order of importance can help me to prioritise the most important things and avoid getting bogged down with the least important.

2. Ask for help. I am so guilty of being too stubborn to ask for help and trying to do everything myself, but something I've had to learn in order to manage my stress levels is ask for help when I need it. Sometimes outsourcing or seeking advice for the things that bring us most stress is all we need to help us find a solution. As the saying goes, 'A problem shared is a problem halved.'

3. Know when to switch off. With the increasing accessibility of social media, we can often feel suffocated by constantly seeing what others are doing, and comparing ourselves to the people we see through the screen on our phones. Try taking some time out and switching your phone off. Going for a walk or reading a book can improve your clarity of thought.

4. Exercise! This can be an excellent stress reliever and is one of the best tools I use to combat stress. Try putting your headphones on, switching your phone on flight mode and train hard – you'll feel a whole lot better for it!

MINDFULNESS

I'm not an expert on this, nor am I going to ask you to meditate daily, recite mantras or do anything crazy. But I will encourage you to just think about incorporating some level of active mindfulness into your week.

So what is mindfulness? Many people describe it as paying more attention than we would normally do to the present moment – to your own thoughts and feelings, and to the world around you – to improve your mental well-being. Even if it does sound a little far-fetched, think about how often you find yourself living your life at a million miles an hour without truly stopping to acknowledge the things around you. When we become more aware of the present moment, we can become more aware of our internal dialogue – and the thoughts and feelings that we experience – giving us more headspace to make sense of these. This heightened sense of awareness can also help us notice signs of stress or anxiety at an early stage, enabling us to deal with them before they develop into bigger issues.

Mindfulness has been so effective in studies that the National Institute for Health and Care Excellence recommends it as a way to help people who have had three or more bouts of depression.

I've listed just a few ways in which you can try to incorporate some form of mindfulness into your week.

1. Notice the everyday. It might sound silly, but allow yourself to become aware of all the things around you. From the weather, nature and the food we eat to the people around us, it can be an extremely powerful experience to increase our awareness of our surroundings, giving a new perspective on life.

2. Breathe. Just taking a few minutes to focus on your breath can be an excellent way to switch off and focus your mind. Try taking deep inhalations through the nose and exhaling out through the mouth, concentrating only on your breath. Close your eyes and take a few minutes to concentrate only on this.

3. Awareness of thought. So many thoughts pass through our mind each day, and how many times do we acknowledge what we are thinking of? Just becoming more aware of what passes through our minds, digesting the information and dealing with each thought, can help us to feel less stressed and more in control of our mental state.

I hope you have more of a tool kit to 360° health and happiness than just good nutrition and exercise. It really is about incorporating as many of these principles into your routine as you need. We are all so unique, and some people may need to work more on this than others, but learning how to use these exercises better equips you to deal with those times in your life when the going does get tough.

PERSONALISING YOUR PROGRAMME

This is the fun bit – once you've tried the workouts in the previous section, you will have a feel for the type of training you enjoy the most. Developing a programme that fits in with both your goals and your lifestyle is key to making progress. In this section I show you how to put together a successful plan and include my personal tips for how to make it work for you.

STEP ONE: DECIDE HOW MANY DAYS YOU ARE REALISTICALLY ABLE TO COMMIT TO TRAINING

Many of us begin our exercise regimes with ambitious ideas of hitting the gym every day, but in reality, for most, this is neither doable nor healthy in the long term. Setting realistic aims for the number of days you are able to commit to training will ensure you don't set yourself up to be disheartened if you cannot work out as much as you'd hoped to.

STEP TWO: DECIDE ON YOUR PREFERRED STYLE OF TRAINING

This can be dependent on a whole host of variables, but it's really important you adhere to your training as much as possible from the outset to get the best results. So, deciding what method of attack you're going to choose before you begin can help to consolidate what you are going to focus your energies on. Have a think about what you are able to do within the time constraints: are you able to

get to the gym or is working out from home more realistic for you? What is your goal, and is there a particular style of training method that will help you progress towards this?

STEP THREE: STRUCTURE YOUR WEEKLY TRAINING SCHEDULE

At this point, you've decided what and how often you are going to work out, and now it's time to bring it all together in your very own programme. Use the table overleaf as a guide, but of course make yours specific to you.

STEP FOUR: KEEP NOTE OF ALL YOUR WORKOUTS, AND TRACK PROGRESSION

To improve and progress, I'd advise keeping track of all your workouts and noting these down so that you can see how you're progressing. Be it reps, sets, rounds of a circuit or weightlifting – the aim is to improve on these week on week to avoid progression plateauing.

AN EXAMPLE OF MY TRAINING WEEK:

I wanted to show you how I put together my training schedule for an example of a week of training. I hope this helps to show you how I structure my own workouts. Feel free to use the table to create your own programme using any of the workouts in this book.

This is, of course, just an example, but it's a good guide to planning your training. I'd advise splitting up your upper- and lower-body workouts to ensure you allow enough time to recover between sessions. See overleaf for my tips on how to ensure progression.

MONDAY	TUESDAY	WEDNESDAY
LOWER BODY	UPPER-BODY PUSH	REST DAY
• Squats • Sumo deadlifts • Bulgarian split squats • Swiss ball hamstring curl • Kettlebell swings	• Push press • Flat bench press • Tricep dips • Spilt-stance single arm arnold press • Pallof press	

Use the table to create your own personalised programme.

* Try my post-workout protein punch on page 55 for a delicious post-workout fuel-up!

THURSDAY	FRIDAY	SATURDAY	SUNDAY
LOWER BODY	**FULL-BODY HIIT**	**UPPER-BODY PULL**	**REST DAY**
• RDLs	• Goblet squats	• Assisted wide grip pull-up	—
• Cable pull-throughs	• Kettlebell clean and press	• Inverted row	
• Reverse barbell lunges	• Reverse lunges w/ kettlebell	• Face pulls	
• Single-leg glute bridges	• Kettlebell swings	• Partial squat single-arm row	
• Staggered stance RDLs	• Kettlebell windmills	• Kneeling single-arm pull-down	
		• Reverse flies	

When I first began training I would use weights a lot lighter than I am able to lift now.

I always advise choosing a weight that challenges you enough to make you feel as though you are fatiguing on the final few reps. Then, aim to improve from this as you progress.

Following a training programme needs consistency. Aim to follow and progress with your plan for at least 8 weeks. See overleaf for progression tips.

HOW DO YOU MAKE REAL PROGRESSION WITH YOUR TRAINING?

When creating your training programme there are some basic principles you need to apply and understand to build a successful personalised programme. Taking some time at the beginning is also often the most overlooked aspect of many training programmes, and can be the main factor in clients becoming disheartened at their lack of progress.

FREQUENCY

It is important to understand that consistency of training is vital. One week of good training is great, but realistically won't make much of a difference to your physique. As well as consistently good nutrition, frequency of training and a good routine are key to a successful exercise programme.

INTENSITY

To really get the most out of this book and your programme, you need to ensure that each training session is of adequate intensity to really challenge you and allow for progression and body change. As previously stated, if you are lifting weights that means choosing a weight that is sufficiently challenging for you, and keeping to strict rest periods to maintain a high heart rate. This also applies to more cardio-based sessions.

VOLUME

Total volume is an equation used by all personal trainers to ensure their clients are getting progressively

stronger, or improving week on week. This can be worked out by multiplying total weight x reps x sets.

An example of this would be squatting 40kg x 8 x 4 which would be the same as 20kg x 16 x 4. You are lifting less weight, but increasing the amount of reps produces the same total output or total volume lifted. This is a useful equation in many circumstances. For example, if you're feeling a little fatigued and want to lift lighter weights, simply increase the number of reps and you will still achieve the same total weight lifted.

This leads me on to the most important factor: a progressive overload. The progressive overload principle states that, in order for a muscle to grow, strength to be gained, performance to increase or for any similar improvements to occur, the human body must be forced to adapt to a tension that is above and beyond what it has previously experienced.

This therefore means that we need to be increasing the demands placed upon the body. Then it will have no other choice but to make the necessary changes and improvements to adapt to this environment and remain capable of performing these tasks.

Whether it's adding an extra rep, increasing the weight, the time the muscle is under tension or simply using something like a resistance band to add more difficulty to an exercise, all of these force the body to adapt and therefore progress. There is no hard-and-fast rule to how often this needs to happen, but I often advise that as soon as an exercise starts to feel easier, or more comfortable, it's time to increase the difficulty.

FREQUENTLY ASKED QUESTIONS

I am asked many questions on a daily basis on my Instagram, so I felt it really important to cover a few of the topics that creep up, and that a lot of people seem to be confused by. With many of these questions, I don't see myself as the all-knowing guru who is averse to anyone else's opinion but my own (an all too common occurrence in the fitness industry). As with anything in life, there will always be various opinions and stances on various topics, and so it's important to keep an open mind and decide in most cases what works best for you, instead of copying exactly what someone else does or says. My most frequently used phrase of late seems to be, 'Just because it worked for one person, does NOT mean it is going to work for the next person.'

HOW MUCH CARDIO SHOULD I DO?

This is probably the most frequently asked question. For those of you who, like me, used to see steady-state cardio as the only form of exercise, it is often perceived that we still need to incorporate cardio into our training to see results. This is, however, totally goal-dependent. Let me explain … If your goal is muscle gain, I wouldn't advise doing much cardio as you want to focus on increasing strength through weight-training, with fewer reps and higher volume of weight lifted. However, if your goal is fat loss, incorporating some cardio into your training (perhaps splitting up weight-training sessions with HIIT workouts twice a week, for example) can help contribute to increasing your daily energy expenditure and help to boost your metabolism and can therefore be beneficial to you achieving your goal. In addition to this, if your goal is, for example, running a marathon, well then of course incorporating cardio into your training is an obvious and necessary choice.

My point is, don't just place a form of exercise into a box. There are many tools of fitness to be used depending on what your specific goal is, so it's important to decide this first and then choose the correct approach accordingly.

CAN I EAT CARBS ON REST DAYS?

Another of the most frequently asked questions. Cutting out carbs simply isn't something I would ever advocate to anyone. Carbohydrates, as I'm sure you know, are our bodies' main source of fuel and energy. Just because you're not training on a given day, doesn't mean that your brain and body don't need any energy to function optimally. I try and keep my eating habits consistent every day, and simply increase carbohydrate intake around my training, but that doesn't mean I exclude carbs on days I don't train and I would really advise you to do the same.

WHAT IS MACRO-TRACKING?

I'm sure many of you have heard this term bandied around on social media of late, but may not actually be sure exactly what it means. Tracking macros is a process by which you track the number of grams of protein, carbohydrates and fats you consume on a particular day. It's a tool often utilised by bodybuilders and physique competitors who have mastered this crazy phenomenon and have no issues about whipping out their food scale at any given moment. For the rest of us, and in reality, it equals restrictive weighing of food, time-consuming measurements and calculations and a diet monitored by an app on your phone.

SHOULD I TRACK MACROS?

If you can't tell from the above, it isn't something I would personally choose to do, nor is it something I advocate to any of my clients. I don't see it as healthy or sustainable, because in reality who wants to be whipping out their phone every time they're hungry to log in said foods details? Not me!

I can totally understand that it may work for some people, but I honestly feel there are other more sustainable and healthy ways to achieve your goal. In my opinion, I just don't see how this instils any sort of healthy habits; instead it leads so many down a dangerous path of obsessive and restrictive eating.

DO I ALWAYS NEED TO WARM UP?

YES! The amount of times I hold my head in my hands when I see people coming into the gym and just start lifting weights completely cold!

To avoid injury, ensure your muscles are sufficiently warm before beginning any exercise. This means incorporating some of the mobility work which I've included at the beginning of the excercise section in this book, too.

DO I NEED TO COOL DOWN?

I would advise, if you have time, to spend around 5-10 minutes cooling down post-workout, particularly if your heart rate has been elevated. This will help prevent things like fainting or dizziness, help to alleviate muscle soreness and allow for the removal of lactic acid which can build up during strenuous exercise.

HOW LONG WILL IT BE UNTIL I SEE RESULTS?

This is something everyone wants to know, but is completely different for each individual. I couldn't put any time-frame on when exactly you will see results, as this comes down to so many variables, from diet and training to hormones, stress levels and genetics. It's worth saying, however, that if you've given it at least 12 weeks of consistent hard work and you're still not seeing results, it might be worth seeing a professional such as a personal trainer or registered nutritionist to see if there might be something going wrong.

I'M WORRIED ABOUT MY FORM – WHAT SHOULD I DO?

If this is something that concerns you, or if you experience pain during any exercise, I would always seek help from a good personal trainer or see a physiotherapist to avoid any injury. Form for me should be at the top of the priority list when it comes to training, so ensuring you are doing an exercise correctly, with the correct posture and alignment and without feeling any sort of niggles or impingements in the body, is paramount.

I'VE GOT AN INJURY. WHAT SHOULD I DO?

If you're struggling with an injury, as frustrating as it may be it's important to take a step back from your training and focus on recovery. Looking after your body is so important; you only get one, so taking a few weeks out in the grand scheme of things really isn't going to affect your long-term goals! If your injury persists, always seek advice from a good physiotherapist and ask them to help with rehabilitation exercise to incorporate into your recovery and rebuild strength in the injured area.

I'VE LOST MOTIVATION. WHAT SHOULD I DO?

First, check out the motivation section of this book, but second, don't beat yourself up. Dips in motivation happen to *all* of us, and getting frustrated at your lack of motivation will only make matters worse. It's sometimes necessary to take a step back and have time away from something before going back and feeling that sense of excitement and motivation that you had when you first started. I often find having a week out helps to reignite my motivation to get back into exercise, but let me assure you: losing motivation is completely normal and you shouldn't stress too much about taking time away from your fitness journey.

IS STRENGTH-TRAINING THE BEST FORM OF TRAINING?

No! Again, many on social media will lead you to believe that strength-training is the be-all and end-all of exercise, and almost look down on those who enjoy any other form of exercise. I personally found my passion in strength-training, but that doesn't mean I don't see the benefits of other forms of training. For me, choosing your form of exercise comes down to two things: what is your goal, and what do you enjoy?

The ultimate aim is to find a way of exercising that you are able to adhere to, so find something you enjoy, as you are then so much more likely to stick to it.

WHAT SHOULD I DO IF I'M STILL SORE TWO DAYS AFTER TRAINING?

Delayed-onset muscle soreness, or DOMS, is pain experienced in your muscles one or two days after you've completed a training session. It is completely normal to experience muscle soreness, and this isn't something you should worry about too much, particularly if you're starting out on your fitness journey. At this point, your muscles probably won't be used to such exertion, but hopefully with time they will adapt and ease as you progress.

While there isn't much you can do to completely alleviate DOMS, there are a few things that can really help ease it, such as taking a bath with some Epsom salts, foam-rolling your muscles to improve blood flow and the breakdown of muscle fascia and ensuring you're adequately hydrated and eating enough protein to support recovery.

DO I ALWAYS NEED TO HAVE A GOAL?

This is something that I think needs to be answered, as it's something I often feel guilty of not having. While I have spent a lot of time in this book helping you understand and build goals, there are times in my own training where I simply want to exercise because I enjoy it, without a specific goal in mind, and this is completely OK, too. Exercise shouldn't always be driven directly by goals. It is social, too, and I often take a class or train with a friend purely for this reason; call it killing two birds with one stone. To say that I am a constantly goal-driven individual would be a complete lie, so while I do find goals really useful in helping me maintain focus and achieve motivation, there are times when I don't have them, too, and I don't think you need to obsess over them if you don't have one right now.

WHAT SHOULD I DO IF I STOP TRAINING FOR A WHILE?

There is no rule about starting and stopping exercise. Sometimes life gets in the way and our training has to take a back seat as other things become prioritised. I've experienced this first hand and my training is often the first thing to go when I get really busy. If you've been out of a routine for a while, there is some chance that you might have decreased a little in strength or stamina, so it's important to understand you won't be able to just pick up from where you left off. However, your body is incredibly resilient, and our muscle memory is excellent, so just stick with it, begin incorporating your training back into your schedule and you'll find it won't be long before you're back on track.

SHOULD I TRUST MY PERSONAL TRAINER?

This is a hot topic of late, with everyone and anyone now able to pay as little as £20 to become a qualified personal trainer. Let me tell you all that simply taking a course to become a personal trainer *does not* make you a personal trainer. I learned how to truly train people while working face to face with clients, day in, day out, being stumped by them and understanding how their bodies work and how best to train each client for their individual needs.

My point is, I hear so many horror stories about personal trainers offering terrible advice, shocking nutritional programmes and just generally shoddy and even dangerous

methods, that I felt it necessary to explain that, just because you've ticked a box and completed an exam, it doesn't make you a credible source of information. Be wary of information given out by PTs. As with any industry, there are some amazing personal trainers, and some not so great ones, and it's important to not believe or not trust everything that they say. A good rule of thumb for me is always to ask a personal trainer to justify why they're giving you an exercise. Anyone can tell someone to bend their knees and squat, but a good personal trainer will be able to justify why they're giving that specific exercise to that specific client and the rationale behind it.

HOW OFTEN SHOULD I TRAIN?

I advise most of my clients to aim for four training sessions a week. I never put a time length on these because, as previously discussed, I believe in quality over quantity. That being said, I know how busy our lives are, and sometimes four sessions can seem ambitious if you've got a busy job, or intimidating if you're a newbie, so don't take this as a hard-and-fast rule. Training as many times as you are able to realistically manage in the long term will benefit you far more than dragging yourself to the gym when you really shouldn't.

Also, to a certain extent, this does depend on your goals and your lifestyle or schedule, but I often think that a good rule of thumb is to aim to train around four to five times a week. I would never really advise training any more than this, as you need to allow time for adequate rest and recovery.

WHAT IS BETTER, CARDIO OR WEIGHT-TRAINING?

This really depends on what your goal is. It would be my advice that if you're aiming for overall fat loss and muscle gain, a combination of both is preferable to really achieve the best results.

I personally like to opt for a combination of the two, basing most of my training sessions around strength and resistance training, with a few HIIT sessions thrown in, too. That way I can ensure I am training my cardiovascular system, helping to boost stamina and promote a boost in metabolism for a prolonged period after exercise, while also building lean muscle through strength-training.

HOW AND WHEN SHOULD I GET STARTED?

This can often be the most daunting part of any journey. My best advice is that there is no better time to start than now. As detailed in my story, I made countless mistakes in my training before I found a way of exercising that worked for me, proving that it isn't just an overnight change.

If you're a complete newbie, I'd advise working your way through the home workout section of this book first, allowing your body to become familiar with all of the movements and acclimatising yourself to training on a regular basis, before progressing on to strength-training. If you've got a little more experience under your belt, I'd suggest jumping straight in with a combination of HIIT training and weight-training if you feel confident enough.

WHY CHOOSE HIIT OVER STEADY-STATE CARDIO?

HIIT isn't the be-all and end-all, but I personally prefer it over steady-state cardio for a number of reasons. First, steady-state cardio is cardiovascular exercise that keeps your heart rate at a constant moderately elevated pace for a sustained period of time. I personally prefer HIIT as it is said to produce results similar to longer, slower cardio workouts in a much quicker time period, therefore making it much more time efficient. It is also arguably more effective at achieving the so-called 'after-burn effect', in which the

metabolism remains elevated for hours, and sometimes even days, after an intense HIIT workout. That being said, if you prefer a long run, swim or walk, both forms of cardio essentially achieve the same thing, in that they help to create a caloric burn. So if HIIT isn't your thing, don't get too hung up on it.

WHAT SHOULD I DO IF I MISS A FEW SESSIONS?

Don't panic! I often get panicked emails or messages from my clients when they miss a session through simple 'life-happens' moments. My response is always – *relax!* You will not undo any of your hard work by missing a few gym sessions and panicking about it will only increase the likelihood that you will then stress and send yourself into a restrictive phase.

Exercise bingeing is a serious condition, and a slippery slope, so being realistic and relaxed about missing training sessions is really important to help develop a balanced approach.

SHOULD I TRAIN IF I'M ILL?

My advice in this situation is to listen to your own body. You know yourself better than anyone, but more often than not, if you're not feeling 100 per cent, then a day of rest can be extremely beneficial to speeding up your recovery. If you are

experiencing a prolonged period of illness or returning to exercise after an illness, I always advise speaking to your doctor before exercising.

HOW DO I CHOOSE A CORRECT WEIGHT FOR MY TRAINING?

This really depends on your goals, but in most cases, and with my own clients, I try and encourage them to lift a weight that is sufficiently challenging for the given rep range, so that by the last few reps they can feel their muscles slightly fatiguing. If you're not experiencing this, you're potentially going a little easy on yourself and could afford to up the weights. If you're struggling from rep one, try reducing the weight to ensure your form remains consistent throughout the set.

CONVERSION CHARTS

DRY WEIGHTS

METRIC	IMPERIAL	METRIC	IMPERIAL
5g	$\frac{1}{4}$oz	500g	1lb 2oz
8/10g	$\frac{1}{3}$oz	550g	1lb 3oz
15g	$\frac{1}{2}$oz	600g	1lb 5oz
20g	$\frac{3}{4}$oz	625g	1lb 6oz
25g	1oz	650g	1lb 7oz
30/35g	1$\frac{1}{4}$oz	675g	1$\frac{1}{2}$lb
40g	1$\frac{1}{2}$oz	700g	1lb 9oz
50g	2oz	750g	1lb 10oz
60/70g	2$\frac{1}{2}$oz	800g	1$\frac{3}{4}$lb
75/85/90g	3oz	850g	1lb 14oz
100g	3$\frac{1}{2}$oz	900g	2lb
110/120g	4oz	950g	2lb 2oz
125/130g	4$\frac{1}{2}$oz	1kg	2lb 3oz
135/140/150g	5oz	1.1kg	2lb 6oz
170/175g	6oz	1.25kg	2$\frac{3}{4}$lb
200g	7oz	1.3/1.4kg	3lb
225g	8oz	1.5kg	3lb 5oz
250g	9oz	1.75/1.8kg	4lb
265g	9$\frac{1}{2}$oz	2kg	4lb 4oz
275g	10oz	2.25kg	5lb
300g	11oz	2.5kg	5$\frac{1}{2}$lb
325g	11$\frac{1}{2}$oz	3kg	6$\frac{1}{2}$lb
350g	12oz	3.5kg	7$\frac{3}{4}$lb
375g	13oz	4kg	8$\frac{3}{4}$lb
400g	14oz	4.5kg	9$\frac{3}{4}$lb
425g	15oz	6.8kg	15lb
450g	1lb	9kg	20lb
475g	1lb 1oz		

568ml = 1 UK pint (20fl oz) | 16fl oz = 1 US pint

LIQUID MEASURES

METRIC	IMPERIAL	CUPS	METRIC	IMPERIAL	CUPS
15ml	½fl oz	1 tbsp (level)	425ml	15fl oz	
20ml	¾fl oz		450ml	16fl oz	2 cups
25ml	1fl oz	⅛ cup	500ml	18fl oz	2¼ cups
30ml	1¼fl oz		550ml	19fl oz	
50ml	2fl oz	¼ cup	600ml	1 pint	2½ cups
60ml	2½fl oz		700ml	1¼ pints	
75ml	3fl oz		750ml	1⅓ pints	
100ml	3½fl oz	⅜ cup	800ml	1 pint 9fl oz	
110/120ml	4fl oz	½ cup	850ml	1½ pints	
125ml	4½fl oz		900ml	1 pint 12fl oz	3¾ cups
150ml	5fl oz	⅔ cup	1 litre	1¾ pints	1 US quart (4 cups)
175ml	6fl oz	¾ cup	1.2 litres	2 pints	1¼ US quarts
200/215ml	7fl oz		1.25 litres	2¼ pints	
225ml	8fl oz	1 cup	1.5 litres	2½ pints	3 US pints
250ml	9fl oz		1.75/1.8 litres	3 pints	
275ml	9½fl oz		2 litres	3½ pints	2 US quarts
300ml	½ pint	1¼ cups	2.2 litres	3¾ pints	
350ml	12fl oz	1½ cups	2.5 litres	4⅓ pints	
375ml	13fl oz		3 litres	5 pints	
400ml	14fl oz		3.5 litres	6 pints	

OVEN TEMPERATURES

All recipes are based on fan-assisted oven temperatures. If you are using a conventional oven, raise the temperature 20°C higher than stated in recipes.

°C	°F	GAS MARK	DESCRIPTION
110	225	¼	cool
130	250	½	cool
140	275	1	very low
150	300	2	very low
160/170	325	3	low to moderate
180	350	4	moderate
190	375	5	moderately hot
200	400	6	hot
220	425	7	hot
230	450	8	hot
240	475	9	very hot

INDEX

Page references in *italics* indicate photographs or illustrations.

ACKNOWLEDGEMENTS

I still can't believe that after two books I am fortunate enough to have had the opportunity to write a third. My first, and most important, thank you therefore goes to you guys, for being the most amazing support and continuing to enjoy what I do. Thank you for purchasing this book, and I hope this in some way gives back to you how much motivation and positivity you give to me. My journey is no different to so many others out there, but what's been so incredible about this life-changing opportunity I've been given is the supportive network of people around me who have made it all possible.

I wouldn't be the person I am, or where I am, without the continued support of my family, who will always be the first people to step in and help when the going gets tough. My mum and dad have been my number one cheerleaders since day one, and I will be forever grateful for all that they do for me. My second thanks goes to Carly, who has been with me since the initial idea of writing a book was suggested over two years, one UK tour, and lots of stressful phone calls ago. She has been my sounding board for ideas, and shared my vision completely for how the books would come together, and I am so grateful to still be lucky enough to work with her.

My editor, Carolyn, and the whole team at HarperCollins; Orlando, Isabel P, Isabel HB, James, and many others behind the scenes have also been the most amazing team an author could wish for. What's stood out is how much fun we have had along the way, and I feel incredibly fortunate to have their continued faith in my ethos and vision. Expanding from this, the amazing team that worked on this particular book, Phil Haynes notably who shot the exercises in this book, as well as Meg Koriat, my lovely make-up artist, also Martin Poole and Kim Morphew and everyone behind the scenes who helped bring the book to life also deserve a huge thanks!

Finally, since moving management this year, my manager Issy has been my absolute rock and the best support anyone could ask for. For me, choosing this career path initially felt like such a huge risk, and whilst as an actress I was so used to slipping on a costume and being someone else on stage, now this was me as me in the spotlight, and knowing that I have constant support and guidance from a manager who just 'gets it' is invaluable.